SUPER**STRETCH**

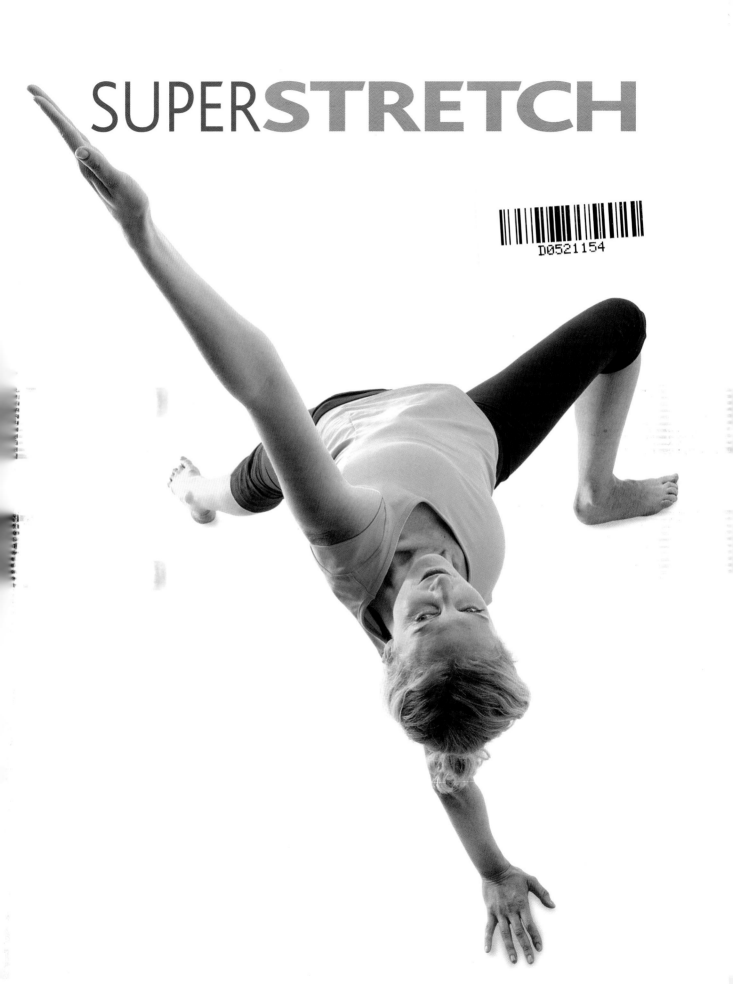

D0521154

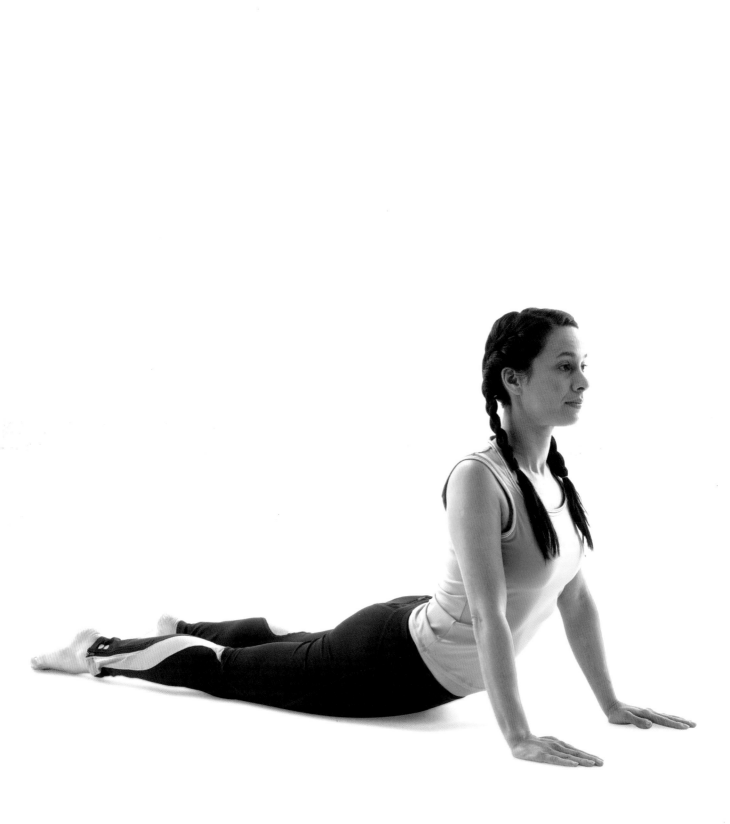

SUPER**STRETCH**

CREATE A LONGER, LEANER, MORE FLEXIBLE BODY IN ONLY 1 HOUR A WEEK!

JACQUELINE LYSYCIA

hamlyn

An Hachette Livre UK Company

First published in Great Britain in 2008 by
Hamlyn, a division of Octopus Publishing Group Ltd
2–4 Heron Quays, London E14 4JP
www.octopusbooks.co.uk

Copyright © Octopus Publishing Group Ltd 2008

Distributed in the United States and Canada by
Sterling Publishing Co., Inc.
387 Park Avenue South, New York, NY 10016–8810

ISBN-13: 978-0600-61703-7

A CIP catalogue record of this book is available from the British Library.

Printed and bound in China

10 9 8 7 6 5 4 3 2 1

CAUTION
It is advisable to check with your doctor before embarking on any exercise
programme. A doctor should be consulted on all matters relating to health and
any symptoms that may require diagnosis or medical attention. While the advice
and information in this book is believed to be accurate and the instructions given
have been devised to avoid strain, neither the author nor the publisher can accept
any legal responsibility for any injury sustained while following the exercises.

CONTENTS

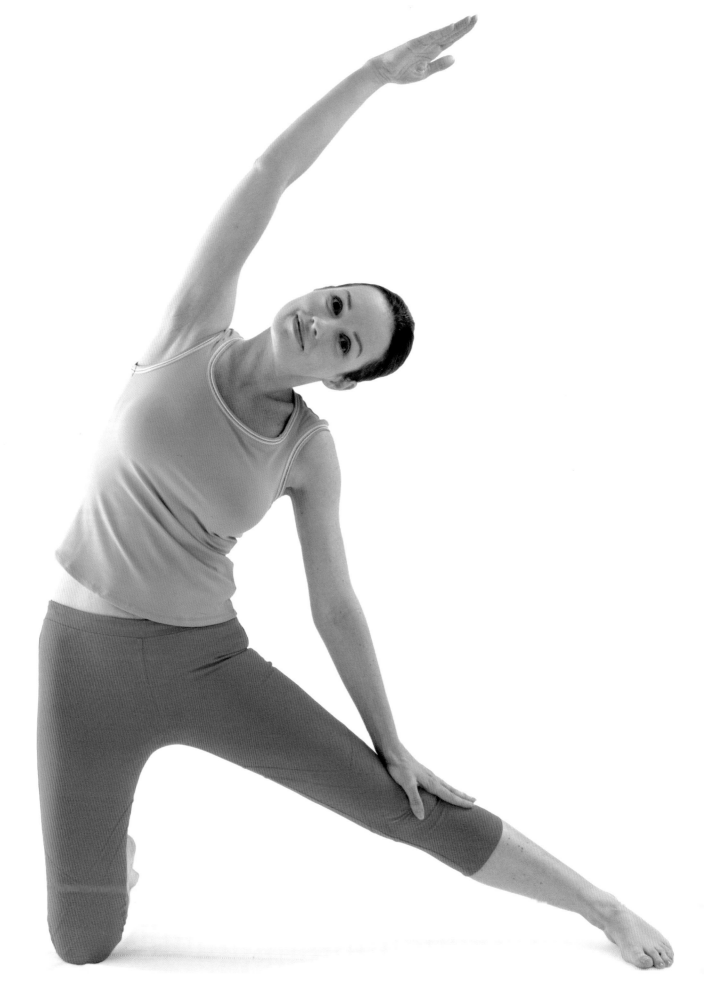

INTRODUCTION

Stretching is a fantastic and easy way to feel good every day. Anyone can benefit from it, and this book will help you get started if stretching is new to you or you want help to develop your technique further.

The selection of stretches covered within the seven chapters have been hand-picked so you can practise and benefit from the most effective stretching techniques in the least amount of time – just one hour each week. Provided you do at least 8–10 minutes of super stretching every day you will be amazed at how energetic you feel, how toned your muscles become and how your flexibility is increased as your muscles and connective tissues are strengthened and rehydrated by vital fluids and nutrients.

The super-stretching techniques have been specifically devised to be effective in a short space of time. The techniques in this book are no ordinary stretches that aim to stretch just one or two muscles – these super stretches stimulate groups of larger muscles to stabilize your body while other muscle groups elongate. The result is a lean, toned and long body that feels great.

There are so many benefits from stretching regularly; your body will love you for it.

why should I do SUPER STRETCHERS?

Stretching regularly will bring life and tone into your muscles and freedom and space to your joints; it will reduce tension and strain in your body; and your spine will feel 10 years younger.

REGULAR STRETCHING WILL:

- Help maintain and improve your flexibility and mobility while energizing the body.
- Lengthen and strengthen your muscles and improve your posture, making you look slimmer and toned.
- Aid the recovery of many common back and neck problems, aches and pains, and help you to avoid them in the future.
- Help prevent injury, pain and strain after exercise and prepare your muscles for movement.
- Increase the range of movement you have around your joints and realign your joints, helping them to function well.
- Improve your skin tone, texture and suppleness.
- Boost your circulation, which helps to make you look and feel younger and more energized.
- Improve your co-ordination and balance by allowing freer and lighter movements.
- Reduces tension and strain in your body caused by work, helping you to relax.
- Support any weight training you do, by reducing post-exercise soreness and enhancing muscle growth while improving your range of movement.

IS SUPER STRETCHING FOR ME?

Stretching is not teaching your body anything new; it is simply awakening your body to what it has forgotten. We are born with amazing suppleness and flexibility, but as the years progress, most of us become less active and stiffness creeps in. Sitting for long periods, working at a desk, carrying a bag on one shoulder, injuries and many other reasons mean that muscles tighten in some areas and weaken in other areas. The problem is that we don't want to recognize what's really happening so we ignore our bodies for as long as possible.

Everyone can learn to stretch, regardless of age, flexibility or physical condition. Stretching is not only for flexible people, in fact, stretching is even more beneficial for people who are very stiff and tight or who have joint or muscle problems.

LOOK YOUNGER, FEEL YOUNGER

Stretching has an anti-ageing effect on your whole body. As we age, the fluid in our body decreases and the elasticity in our muscles, connective tissues, tendons, ligaments and skin start to weaken; we literally start to shrink. Gravity doesn't help the situation.

When you stretch you are helping your body to remain young as it boosts the circulation of lubricating fluid and blood to these vital areas, so they stay supple and strong. Your face and skin also start to show signs of ageing, but stretching helps to stimulate and nourish your face, helping you to look alert and energized. Stretching also helps to improve your posture, helping you to move and breathe easily, and look dynamic.

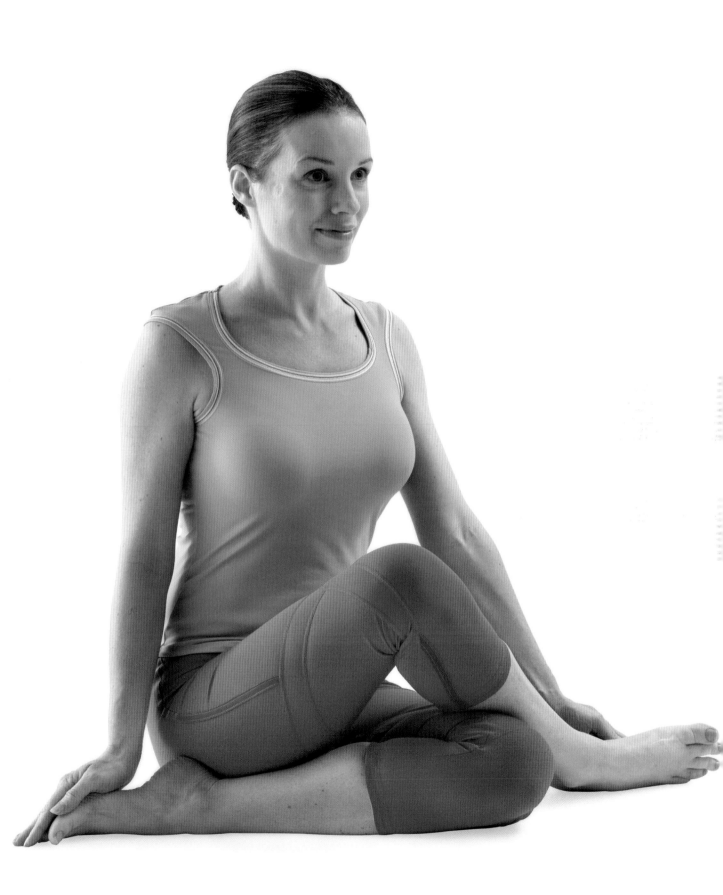

the BENEFITS of STRETCHING

Whether you want to improve your sports performance, reduce your risk of injury, improve your posture or alleviate existing aches and pains, you will benefit from stretching.

Stretching keeps your muscles supple, prepares you for movement and helps you make the transition from inactivity to activity without undue strain on your body. It is really important to stretch before and especially after you exercise to help protect your body from injury. Stretching when your muscles are warm is also a good time to extend your range of movement. Not stretching after exercise can lead to muscle tightness, inflexibility and muscle strain.

IMPROVE YOUR POSTURE

We are born with good posture, and with our bodies balanced and ready for movement. As we age, gravity, lack of mobility and doing repetitive tasks such as driving or carrying a bag on one shoulder, can lead to imbalance in muscle strength around the body. This can lead to poor posture, for example, if your shoulder muscles are tight, this can lead to hunching your back. Weak abdominal muscles can lead to lower back pain, as the back muscles struggle to support the area. Stretching will help you to improve your posture as it strengthens your muscles in a balanced way, working on both sides of the body.

RAISE YOUR BODY AWARENESS

Following the stretches in this book will help you to become more aware of your body. You will discover where your strengths and weaknesses are, and where your body has been under strain. If you find some of the stretches challenging or a little uncomfortable, it means that they have found a tight spot in you, and that your body is really benefiting from doing the

stretch. Other stretches will simply be a breeze and your body will release feel-good endorphins that will put you in a great mood.

Your breathing rate will change to accommodate the different stretches and it is important you listen to your breath as it tells you the state of your nervous system. If your breath becomes fast and won't slow down while in the stretch, then the stretch may be too challenging for you, at the moment. Your body knows exactly what is nourishing and harming it. All you have to do is reacquaint yourself with your body and act accordingly.

Stretching is peaceful, relaxing and non-competitive. All the exercises in this book can be modified to suit you, and you are the one in control. Super stretching gives you the freedom to be yourself and enjoy being yourself through feeling good; it relaxes your mind as well as your muscles. I hope that you will learn more about your body and be able to develop to your own potential, with an enjoyment of stretching and movement that will last a lifetime.

Caution
- Don't push your body to the threshold of serious discomfort and pain. If you start to shake, then you have taken the stretch too far.
- If you have a pre-existing condition or illness consult your doctor before attempting the stretches in this book.

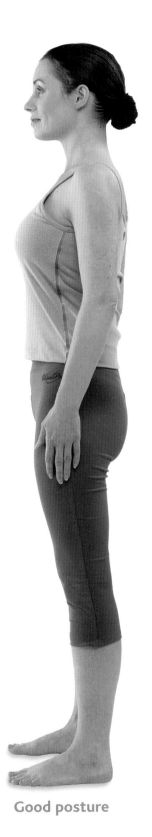

Good posture

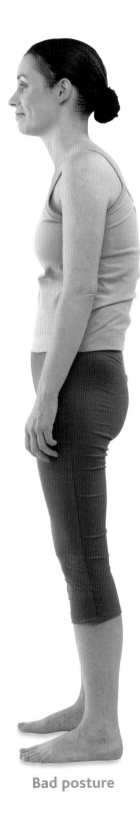

Bad posture

STRETCHING TO RELAX AND FEEL GREAT

Stretching stimulates the brain to release 'feel-good' hormones, including serotonin. This is released by glands and then spreads throughout your body, which nourishes your organs and muscles, and makes you feel energized and positive. Your body and mind feel relaxed and your heart rate and blood pressure stabilize. This is one reason why it is so important to stretch when working; it gives you time to relax and re-energize your body and mind.

When you stretch specific parts of the body, such as your spine, your brain also triggers the release of chemicals that are specific to that area, for example, cerebral spinal fluid. If we led more active, mobile lives, our daily activities would ensure that our bodies received these vital fluids more frequently. As this is not the case for many of us, stretching helps to keep our bodies feeling active and functioning as they were designed to.

Stretching helps to pacify our nervous system by releasing chronic tension trapped between the fine layers of muscle and small bones and joints. Chronic tension held in the body over long periods of time can cause premature ageing and this can create feelings of heaviness in the physical body. When our brains relax through the stretching of our physical body, it sends out an anti-ageing signal for cell renewal. Therefore, stretching can also help to maintain a youthful self.

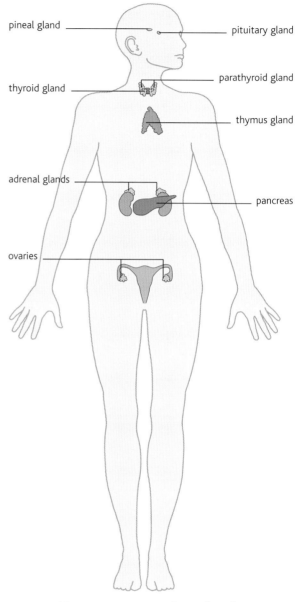

Hormone secreting glands

MASSAGING YOUR INTERNAL ORGANS

Twisting, bending and stretching our bodies also massages inside, especially the vital organs and glands contained in the torso area such as the liver, kidneys, intestines, pancreas and adrenal glands.

Stretching is a gentle, safe way to stimulate your organs and stimulate the supply of blood and nutrients to them. It can also help your organs to perform their function, by helping to remove away waste and toxins in the blood supply. Massaging your intestines when you twist also helps your digestion by aiding food to progress and keeping the intestines supplied with fresh blood. Your pancreas is designed to control your blood sugar levels, so a stretch that massages this area can help to calm you.

The deep, relaxed breathing that you experience when stretching helps your organs to function more effectively by releasing more toxins out of your body each time you exhale.

The chapter *Gentle therapeutic stretches* contains stretches that are designed specifically to massage your organs, as well as stretching muscles and connective tissue. This is especially important if you feel tired or a little unwell as it can help your body to function well. The stretches are gentle and ideal for those occasions when you don't have very much energy. However, most of the stretches in the book will also benefit the inside of your body.

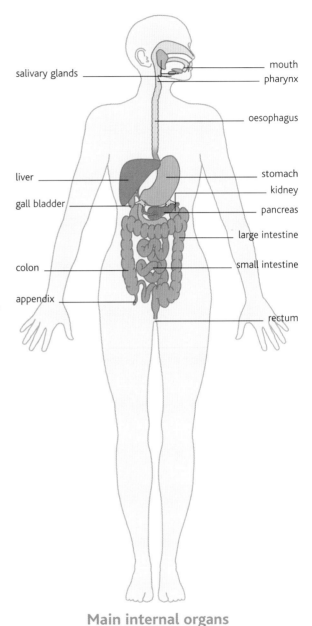

Main internal organs

WHAT HAPPENS
when you stretch

The stretches in this book target areas of the body that tend to need stretching most, such as the spine and back, neck, shoulders, hips and legs.

When stretching you mobilize muscles, the muscles around a joint, and connective tissues, such as ligaments and tendons. Connective tissue holds together all the elements of our bodies, such as bones, organs and muscles. It also supplies nutrients and energy around the body.

As you stretch you will feel the 'pull' of your muscles and tissues away from your bones. This action helps the muscles and tissues to fill with vital fluids and nutrients, which helps to keep them lubricated, supple and strong.

STRETCHING YOUR JOINTS

Shoulders, neck, knees and hips are joint areas where many of us feel discomfort or pain, and are areas where we can all benefit from stretching regularly. Your joints are connected to your bones and muscles with connective tissue. This can become dry and brittle as we age becoming less and less elastic, causing stiffness and pain. The stretches in the book will help you to soften the connective tissue around your joints.

When stretching and softening a joint, stretch very slowly to avoid injury and to let your body get used to the feelings. You can expect to feel some major increases in the range of movement of your joints within three weeks of starting this programme. After around five weeks you will feel taller, more flexible and relaxed. You will also notice you have more energy as your body moves freely with less effort.

STRETCHING YOUR MUSCLES

Every muscle in your body has a different threshold so be aware of how you feel when you stretch. Identify any tightness and aim to challenge these areas without pushing yourself to pain. Never 'bounce' into a stretch and instead follow each step carefully and take your time. Notice if you are being complacent, and also notice if you are being aggressive. Stay relaxed and simply focus your attention on the muscle being stretched. This book includes light, medium and developmental stretches. Start with the light stretches. Within 5 minutes of super stetching your body will respond according to how you feel.

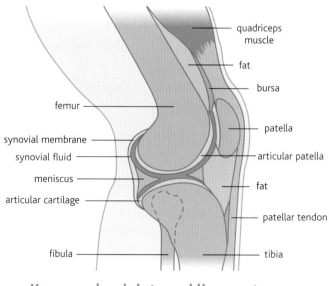

quadriceps muscle

fat

bursa

femur

patella

synovial membrane

articular patella

synovial fluid

meniscus

fat

articular cartilage

patellar tendon

fibula

tibia

Key muscles, joints and ligaments

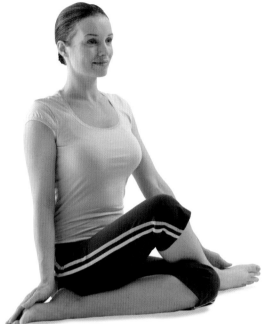

A light stretch

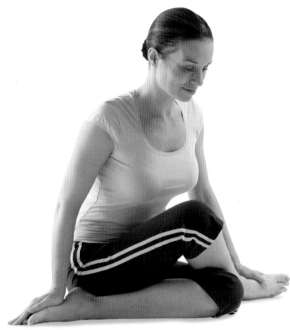

A medium stretch

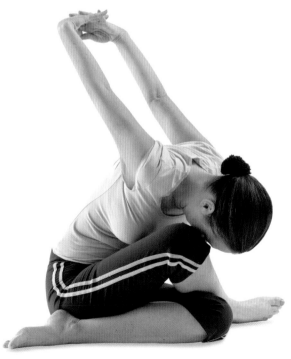

A developmental stretch

A light stretch

When you first engage a muscle you may feel a gentle 'lengthening' feeling. This type of stretch will not develop your flexibility, but it does feel good and you relax in the stretch for a while to help relax the muscle. As you develop your stretching technique you will become aware of a 'letting go' zone in each stretch. This is the point at which you relax and let your muscles lengthen.

A medium stretch

This borders on feeling slightly uncomfortable but not painful. A medium stretch helps to lengthen your muscle a little.

A developmental stretch

Challenging and can be uncomfortable but not painful. Your muscle will be lengthening quite a bit. There is a fine line between discomfort and pain so it may take you a while to recognize your threshold.

WHEN TO stretch

Stretching can be done at any time of the day that you feel works for you. You can stretch at home, at work, after exercise, for five minutes or for an hour. Stretch when you feel like it; if you feel stiff or have been standing or sitting for a long time, you will benefit from stretching for a few minutes. If you are working you may want to do a few stretches throughout the day to alleviate tension or to help you re-energize.

FINDING THE TIME TO STRETCH

The super-stretch programme recognizes that in our modern world we don't have much spare time, so included in this book are only the most beneficial stretches that can be done in the minimum amount of time. All the stretches can be done at home, with no equipment, and many can be done at work or in the gym, in fact, whenever you need to stretch to relieve tension or relax tired muscles. The great news is that you can do a super-stretch programme in just 10 minutes a day, and if you manage this on most days of the week, you will really notice the benefits.

Experts believe that we should stretch twice a day for the maximum and fastest benefits. It will be great if you can stretch in the morning and again in the evening. Five minutes each time is all that is required, but sometimes you may only have time to do two or three stretches, and that is a good start.

If you have a specific area of the body that needs work, try to dedicate more time to your stretching.

TIP

Aim to stretch a little every day. Stretching for just 5–10 minutes a day you will see benefits, and more than 10 minutes even greater benefits. Once stretching becomes part of your day you will probably want to spend longer practising, even staying in positions for significant lengths of time.

For example, if you have a groin strain and your physiotherapist has instructed you to focus on elongating your hamstrings, aim to complete *Stretching your hips, legs and spine* each day – you will save yourself some money, too!

A DAILY ROUTINE

If you have time to spend longer on the super-stretch programme, and want to stretch every day, choose a time in the day when you feel warm and relaxed. Bear in mind that stretching in the morning is generally more uncomfortable as your body has been still overnight. If this is your only time to stretch then take it easy, and move gently in and out of the positions. Look out for the stretches in the programme that are ideal for getting started in the morning and really boost the circulation.

If you stretch in the afternoon or evening, your body will be warmer from the day's activities and the stretches will feel more comfortable. This can be a good time to try something new and more challenging.

HOW TO stretch

Each stretch is explained clearly, with step-by-step photographs to help you stretch correctly. Here are a few points to help you get the most from your stretching.

BREATHING WHILE YOU STRETCH

Yoga and Pilates require very specific breathing, but when stretching, your breathing can be very easy and natural. All the stretches should be performed with your most natural breath.

Try not to control your breath in any way; simply allow your body to inhale and exhale. Breathe through your nose, and as you inhale you will take in fresh oxygen and as you breathe out, you will dissipate toxins.

I give guidelines during the exercises on how and when to move when you inhale and exhale. Generally, you inhale and pause a stretch, and as you exhale, you move a little deeper into the stretch. Trying to move or stretch more as you breathe in can feel uncomfortable; when you exhale, you create space within your body. Always gently float into the stretch on the breath out; your breath will feel more natural and you will find the stretch easier to perform.

In the *Dynamic stretches*, you may find that your breathing will speed up a little, and this is a healthy sign that your body is working and warming up.

Breath cycles

Each breath in and out is called a 'breath cycle'. One inhalation and the stillness afterwards, and one exhalation and the stillness afterwards is one breath cycle. I give guidelines on how many breath cycles to hold each stretch for, but if you want to remain in the stretch for longer or to finish sooner, then listen to your body. You are the only one who knows what your body feels like, so be kind and honest to yourself.

Lengthen your tailbone

Your tailbone (also known as 'sacrum') is located at the base of your spine and between your hip bones. When asked to 'lengthen your tailbone' aim to lift your front hip bones upwards so your tailbone lengthens downwards. Try not to tuck your tailbone under or tighten your buttocks. Broaden through the balls of your feet and draw your thigh muscles into your thigh bones to stabilize the tailbone lift. This position realigns your pelvis.

Keep your abdomen empty

When you inhale and fill your ribcage, you will feel an upward lift in your upper trunk, creating more space in your abdomen. As you exhale, try to maintain the length and feel the emptiness in your abdomen. Try not to suck your stomach in as your breathing will become shallow and you will lock tension into your body.

Maintain a strong core

When you inhale and broaden your ribcage, maintain this broadening and lengthen your abdomen so that your 'core' remains strong in all the stretches. This is an important part of super stretching.

Additionally, a strong core helps you to train your spine and abdominal muscles, and the strength of your core muscles is super important for maintaining the health of your spine, which carries you into your older years.

GETTING started

You do not need any special equipment or clothing to stretch and you can stretch anywhere, for example, at your desk, in the garden or at the gym.

If you want to work through a programme of stretches from this book at home, these tips will help you feel comfortable:

- Find an area where you have space to sit or lie down and move your arms about.
- Check that you cannot slip on the floor; use a mat if you have one.
- Take your shoes and socks off and stretch with bare feet.
- If you plan to try some of the more challenging stretches, wear something loose, cool and stretchy.
- A rolled up towel or cushion can be useful to make some of the stretches more comfortable.
- Switch off your phone and focus on your body.

I recommend that you always begin with the warm-up stretches on pages 22–34. It is important to prepare your body every time with warm up stretches, as they increase circulation in your blood supply and loosen up your joints. This helps to make the most of your stretching session

If you have time, move on to the next chapter, *Dynamic Stretches*. As you progress, you can use some of the dynamic stretches as warm-ups. All the stretches are easy to manage if you follow the step-by-step instructions and listen to what your body is telling you. Then choose one or two of the other chapters, according to the area of your body you would like to focus on, or choose two or three stretches from each chapter to give you a balanced, all-

over stretch. Some of the stretches are ideal as a 'cool-down' at the end of a stretching session, so add one of these to relax your body.

Super stretching is easy, but it is important to read the book carefully and follow the exercise techniques correctly. If rushed, or if you push your body too far, you could do more harm than good.

THE PROGRAMME

The exercises within this book have been split into seven sequences including warm-ups and stretches that focus on key problem areas of the body:

- Warm-up stretches.
- Dynamic stretches.
- Stretching your spine.
- Stretching your hips and legs.
- Stretching your hips, legs and spine.
- Stretching your upper body.
- Gentle therapeutic stretches.

If you are feeling energetic you can warm up and practise the dynamic stretches followed by another body section or a few techniques from each section. Try to vary your programme as much as possible and aim to set aside at least 10 minutes every day.

If you are feeling less energetic or are recovering from illness, do the warm-up stretches and then focus on the gentle therapeutic stretches on pages 112–23. This is a great section for massaging your internal organs and softening connective tissue, so afterwards you feel energized.

TIP

If you are pressed for time, do the warm-up stretches and choose one or two stretches from another chapter to stretch an area of your body that feels tight today.

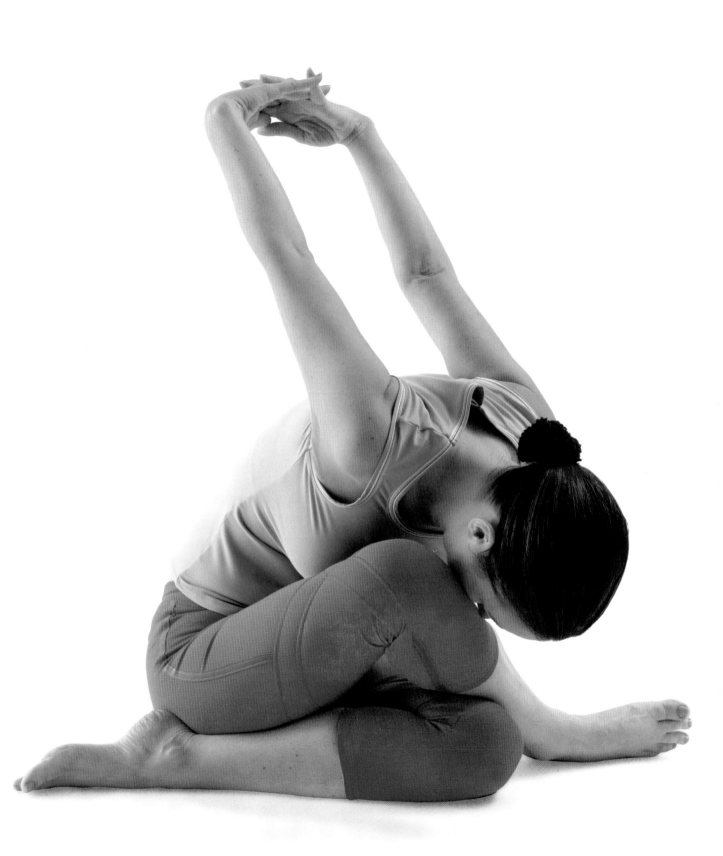

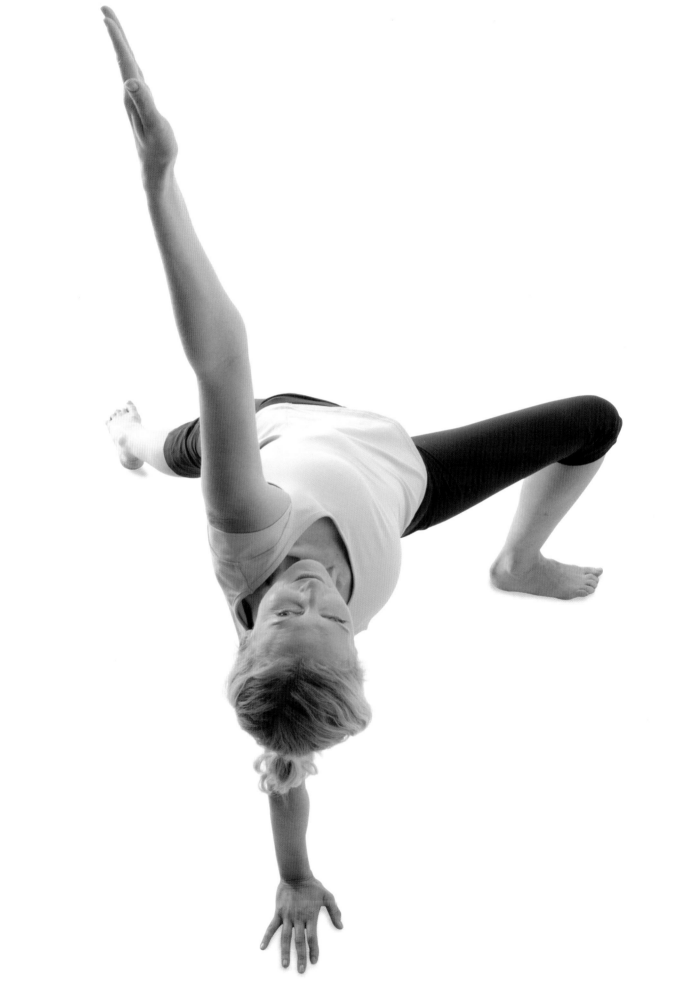

WARM-UP STRETCHES

The stretches in this chapter have been developed to warm up your joints and muscles in the minimum amount of time. Working through the programme will also help to *energize* your body, and help you to get moving in the morning or prepare you for exercise.

The programme will take just a few minutes and it is important that you keep moving and breathe deeply to promote internal body heat and increase the circulation of body fluids (see page 12). Take time over the routine and do not push into any stretch aggressively; listen to your body and be aware that too much too soon could lead to injury.

It is important to relax and 'let go' during the stretches. This helps to release any tension in your body. Sometimes we do not realize we are doing it, but we hold tension all the time. Our muscles have a certain level of tension to ensure we function correctly; however, when we are stressed, angry, tired or have been working too hard, our bodies can hold onto stress on a deep, physical level. Once you have learned how to relax, you will discover a 'relax and let go' zone during every stretch.

THIS SECTION INCLUDES 14 WARM-UP SUPER STRETCHES:

STANDING side bend

This stretch lengthens your spine and waist and relaxes your shoulders. It also targets the IT band muscle that runs down the side of your hips and thighs, helping to increase your mobility and flexibility.

LENGTHEN YOUR TAILBONE

To 'lengthen your tailbone' lift your front hip bones upwards so your tailbone lengthens downwards. Try not to tuck your tailbone under or to tighten your buttocks. This movement realigns your pelvis.

1 Place your left hand on your left hip. Cross your right foot over your left foot. Lengthen your tailbone as you inhale and stretch your right arm up. Exhale and lean into your left hip. **Hold for 4–5 breath cycles.** Repeat on the other side. **Repeat the exercise 10 times.**

stretch

ARM RELEASE swing

This is a great moving stretch technique to dissipate tension from your shoulders and neck that builds up with computer work or jobs that involve constant lifting of the arms. Leaving tension to build can lead to headaches.

BREATHING OUT

When you inhale, you will feel an upwards lift in your upper trunk, creating more space in your abdomen. As you exhale, try to maintain the length in your abdomen and feel the emptiness in your lower trunk.

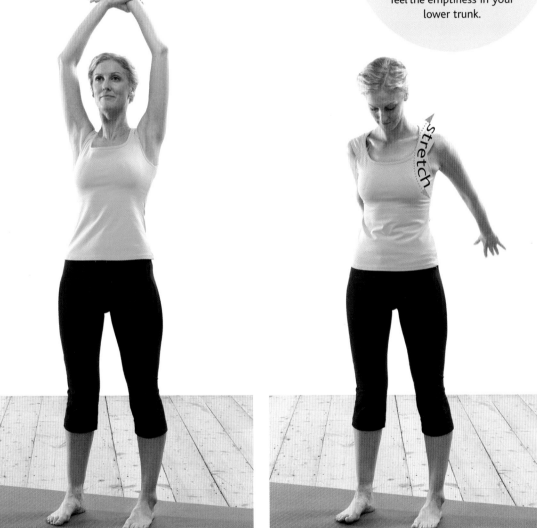

1 Stand with your feet hip-width apart. Inhale and extend both arms above your head. Keep your tailbone long and your abdomen empty as you exhale. Your knees should be slightly soft and your elbows loose. Cross your wrists above your head.

2 Inhale and, as you exhale, swing your arms down and behind you. **Repeat the swing down and up 15 times.** Maintain control and keep your spine and pelvis in alignment. Use a strong breath; inhale deeply and exhale slowly, taking longer on the exhale.

LEG LUNGE twist

This stretch opens your hips and lengthens the psoas muscles located in the hips, which if left to tighten can lead to lower back pain. This is a useful stretch to prepare you for exercise.

TIP

Your front leg should be at a 90° angle to the floor throughout this stretch.

1 Stand with your feet hip-width apart and place your hands on your hips. Inhale and step forward with your left leg into a lunge. Exhale and straighten your back leg, pressing your right hip down towards the floor. Inhale and exhale to lengthen your tailbone and look forwards.

stretch

2 Keeping your balance, inhale and extend your right arm forwards and your left arm back. With your arms in a parallel line, exhale and twist gently to the left. Look in the direction of the twist. **Hold for 5–10 breath cycles. Repeat 3–5 times**, then repeat on the other side.

stretch

BEND and EXTEND

A good stretch to release any tension in your lower and upper back. It also targets the hamstring muscles in the backs of your legs. If you play sport or wear shoes with a heel this technique will lighten the legs and soften the back.

CAUTION

If you have a back injury or a weak back, keep your knees slightly bent when in position 2.

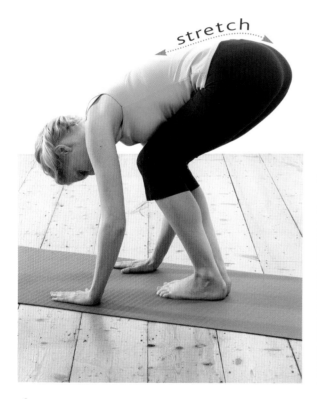

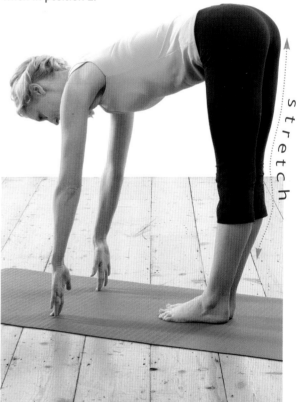

1 Stand with your feet together and inhale to fill your ribcage. As you exhale, draw your abdomen into towards your spine and bend forwards at the hips. Aim to place your hands flat on the floor; bend your knees as much as necessary.

2 Inhale and lengthen your spine while coming onto your fingertips. Exhale as you bend your knees and bring your palms flat to the floor again. Keep your heels down. **Repeat 10 times**, increasing the range of movement each time, using your breath.

HIP circle

Your hips can store a great deal of tension, which can manifest itself in backache and general stiffness. This movement improves mobility in your hips and helps to relieve tension throughout your body.

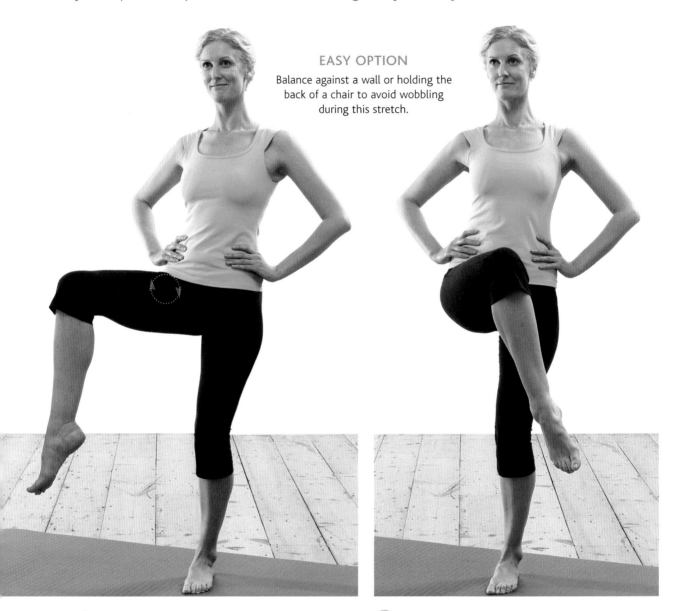

EASY OPTION
Balance against a wall or holding the back of a chair to avoid wobbling during this stretch.

1 Stand with your feet hip-width apart and your hands on your hips. Inhale to fill your ribcage – press your hands slightly into your hips to help elevate your ribcage. As you exhale, lift your right knee while keeping your spine extended.

2 Inhale to fill your lungs and as you exhale, make a 'figure of 8' shape with your raised leg, working from your hip. Keep the movement smooth, alternating between the inhale and the exhale. **Repeat 5 times**, then repeat with the other leg.

SPINE roll

A good stretch to realign the spine curvature and lengthen the hamstrings. It can be done throughout the day; rolling down your spine helps to release any tension trapped between your vertebrae.

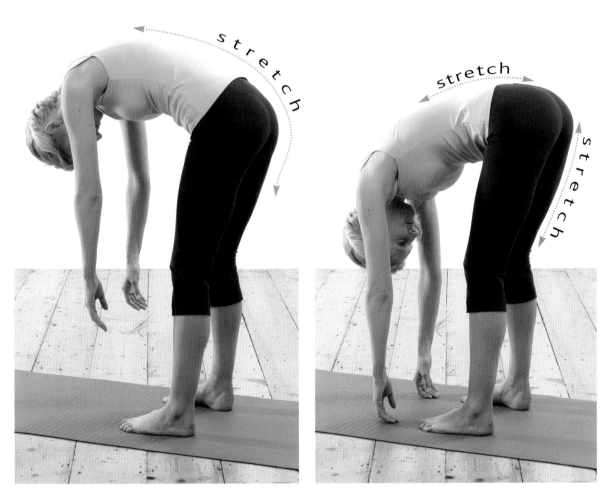

1 Stand with your feet hip-width apart, with a slight bend in your knees and your arms hanging by the sides of your body. Inhale to fill your lungs and as you exhale, slowly begin to curl towards the floor, vertebra by vertebra.

2 Pause when you run out of breath, breathe in, then continue to roll down as you exhale. Keep your abdomen drawn into your spine. **When you reach as far as you can, hang in this position for a few breath cycles.** Inhale and exhale to roll up slowly to standing.

LEG swing back

A moving stretch that helps to soften your hips, improving their mobility, increasing circulation and toning your thighs. It warms and relaxes your legs and reduces any swelling caused by standing for long periods. It also helps to improve balance.

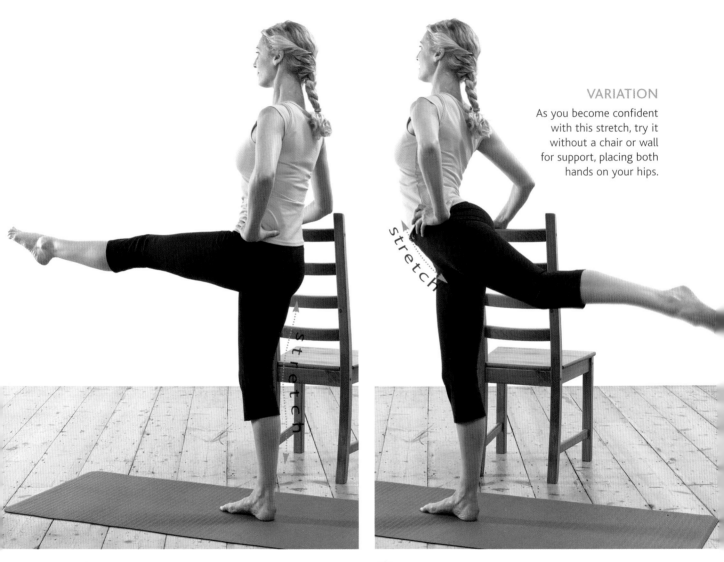

VARIATION

As you become confident with this stretch, try it without a chair or wall for support, placing both hands on your hips.

1 Place one hand on a chair or wall for support and the other on your hip. Lengthen through your spine. Inhale and, as you exhale, gently swing your outer leg forwards to release the hip area.

2 Inhale and, as you exhale, swing your leg gently behind you. **Repeat 15 times,** building up the rhythm of the movement. Rotate your toes gently outwards as you swing and feel the weight of your leg come down with your foot. Repeat with the other leg.

HEAD to KNEE hug

This stretch releases any tightness in your hips and legs and increases circulation in the spine and pelvis. It also stretches the spine deeply and helps to improve posture and balance.

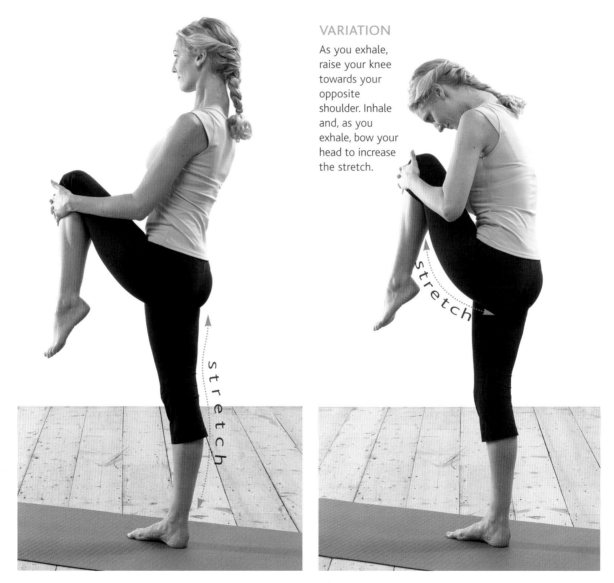

VARIATION

As you exhale, raise your knee towards your opposite shoulder. Inhale and, as you exhale, bow your head to increase the stretch.

1 Stand on your right leg and balance carefully. Inhale and raise your left knee towards your chest. Exhale and lengthen your abdomen to support your spine.

2 Lengthen your tailbone and bow your head towards your knee. **Hold this stretch for 3 breath cycles. Repeat 10 times**, then repeat with the other leg.

NECK stretch

Most of us have experienced tension in our neck and shoulders. This stretches the upper trapezius muscle located between your neck and shoulders, which is responsible for elevating your shoulders, tilting your head and rotating your chin.

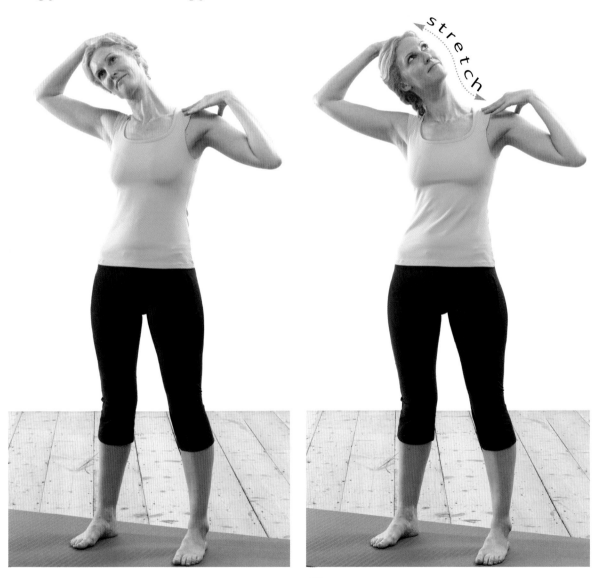

stretch

1 Place your left hand on your left shoulder. Place your right hand on your head, just above your left ear. Inhale, and as you exhale, gently allow the weight of your right arm to pull your head down towards your right shoulder.

2 Maintaining the gentle stretch in the left side of your neck, slowly inhale and, as you exhale, turn your chin towards your left shoulder and upwards. **Hold for 3 breath cycles**, then repeat on the other side. **Repeat as many times as you feel comfortable.**

the SAW stretch

An effective stretch that takes the spine through a twisting movement. Rotating your spine is beneficial as you soften out any stiffness from sitting facing forwards for long periods.

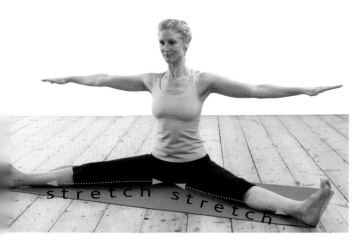

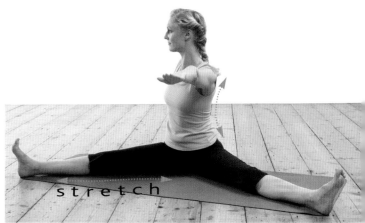

1 Sit on the floor with your legs extended in a straddle position with your knees flat on the floor and feet flexed. Extend your spine upwards and draw your abdomen in towards your spine. Inhale and exhale to extend both arms out to your sides, keeping your shoulders relaxed.

2 Inhale and rotate to the right, keeping your spine tall and long.

3 As you exhale, reach your left arm towards your right foot as your right arm rotates behind you. Aim to reach to your big toe. Return to sitting and inhale. Exhale and reach to the other side. **Repeat 10 times**, keeping the movement continuous.

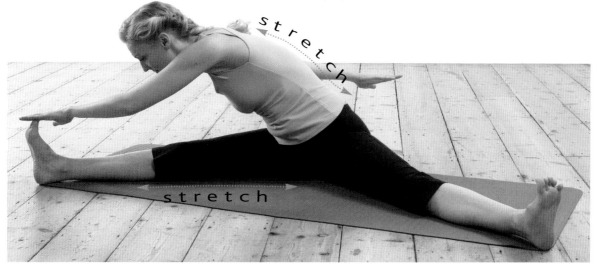

EASY twist

This stretch opens the tailbone area (also known as *sacrum*) and releases tension in the hips that can lead to back pain. It also lengthens the outer hip joint, releasing tension that can build up from lack of movement.

1 Lie on your back with your knees bent and your feet hip-width apart and flat on the floor. Place your arms on the floor level with your shoulders, palms facing the ceiling.

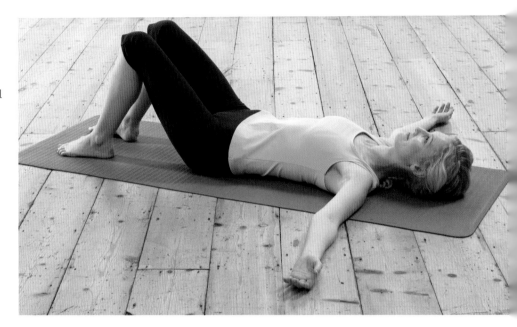

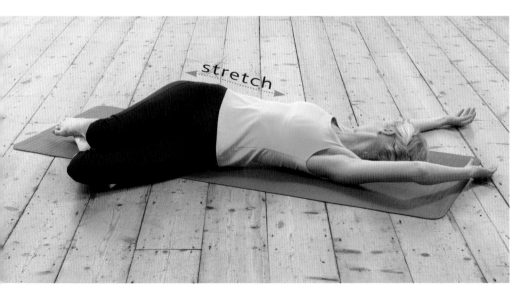

stretch

2 Inhale and, as you exhale, allow your legs to roll to the left. Take your arms and head to the right. **Rest here for 3–5 breath cycles,** then repeat on the other side.

ARM POSITION

If you prefer, take your arms above your head and just move your knees. You may find this position is more comfortable.

HIP and SPINE softener

A great opener for your hips and spine, and the muscles that connect them. This area can become very tight in adults causing back pain, so it is important to stretch it regularly.

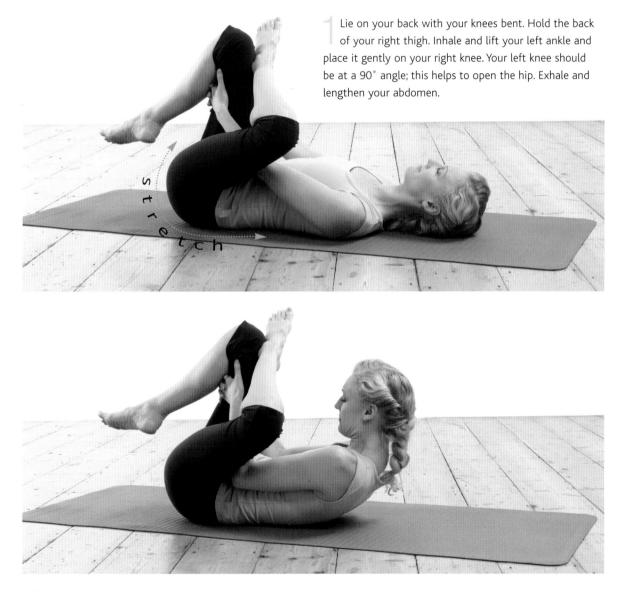

1 Lie on your back with your knees bent. Hold the back of your right thigh. Inhale and lift your left ankle and place it gently on your right knee. Your left knee should be at a 90° angle; this helps to open the hip. Exhale and lengthen your abdomen.

stretch

2 Inhale and curl the upper spine up from the floor. Exhale and curl your spine back to the floor. **Repeat 10 times**, then repeat on the other side. Aim to increase the movement gently with each cycle.

KNEELING stretch

A simple stretch that can be used to relax and for meditation. Try to focus internally; the more you practise kneeling, the more you will recognize the changing sensations inside your body as you stretch.

PELVIS POSITION

Adopt a neutral position that feels comfortable in the lower back; it should not be pushed forwards or backwards causing the lower back to round.

1 Place a towel under your bottom and kneel comfortably. Rest the backs of your hands on your thighs. Be aware of your breathing; your ribcage expands as you inhale, and your abdomen is long and empty as you exhale. **Rest in this position for 1–5 minutes.**

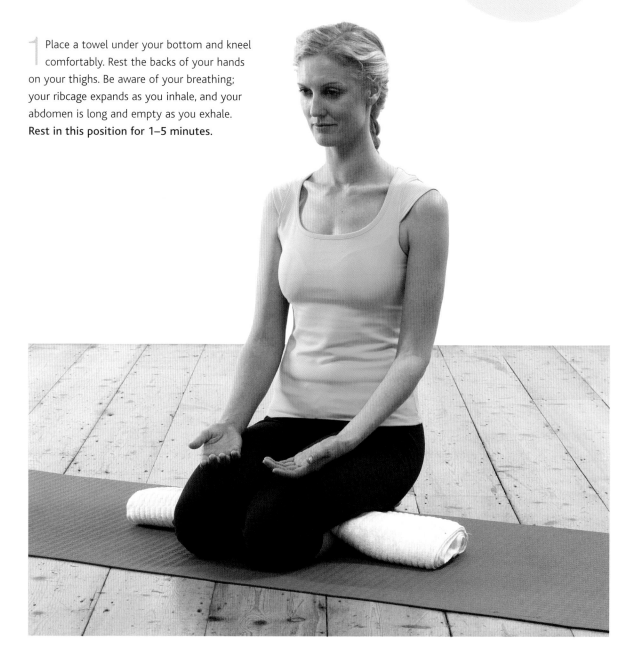

the PENTACLE

A relaxation technique that is ideal for the end of a stretching session. It helps you to identify how it feels when you let your body relax. Aim to *soften* your body from inside right through to your skin.

TIP

Try to feel the changing sensations of *chi*, moving in and out of the parts of the body that were stressed in any previous stretches. *Chi* is energy flow around the nervous system that governs mood, self-esteem and the correct functioning of the glands and internal organs.

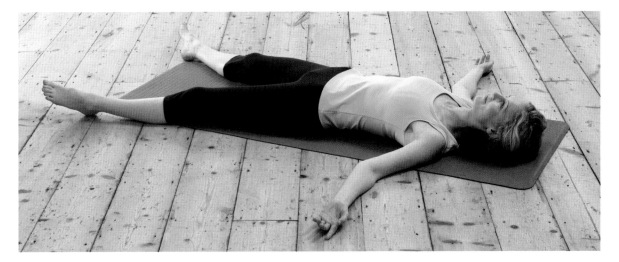

1 Lie on the floor, with your arms and legs spread out in a star shape. Make sure your lower spine does not arch away from the floor; if it does, bend your legs and rest your feet flat on the floor. Close your eyes and let go of any tension. **Rest in this position for 1–5 minutes.**

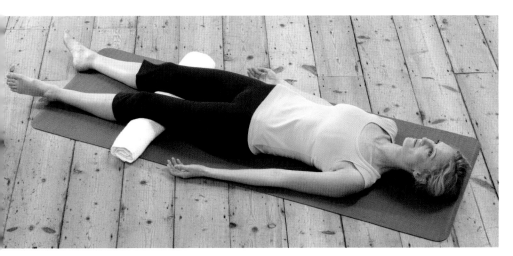

VARIATION

If your spine feels uncomfortable in this position, place a rolled towel underneath the back of your knees to release the lower back.

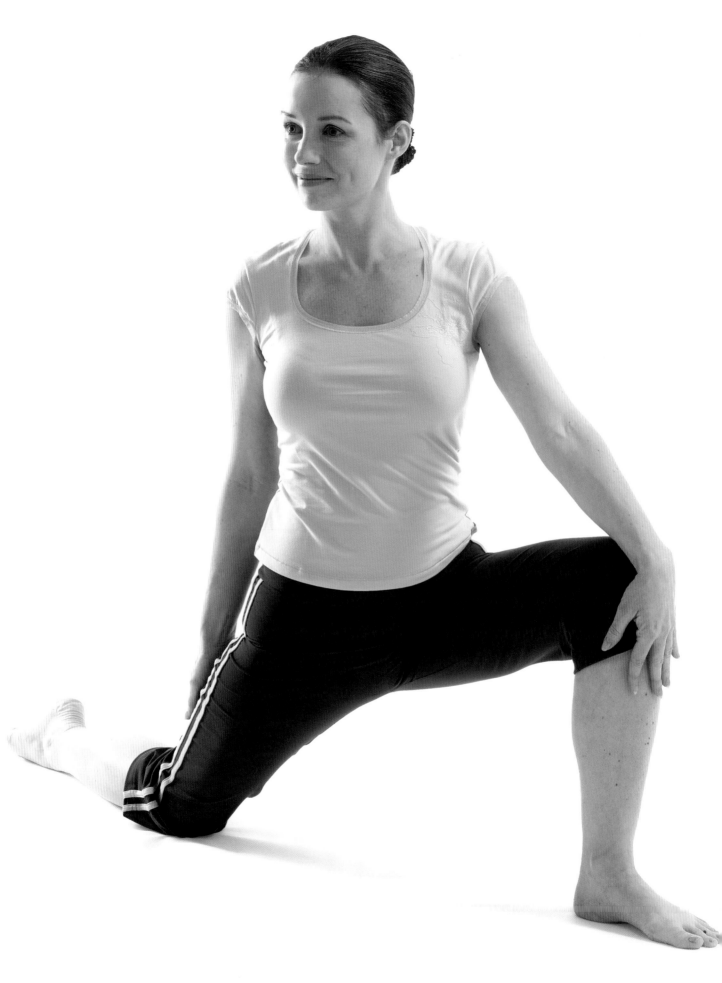

DYNAMIC STRETCHES

This group of stretches is challenging and dynamic. It is designed to be done as a complete sequence, to energize you and prepare you for using your body to its full potential. The stretches are best performed after completing the warm-up stretches (see pages 20–34).

The dynamic stretches use bigger muscle groups and can feel more challenging than other stretches, but they are great for improving circulation and increasing the range of movement around your joints. The stretches are fluid and you may need to practise them individually before attempting the whole group. Focus on your muscles and take your time as you stretch.

As a whole, this chapter is a great sequence to do to wake up your body in the morning or mid-afternoon. Practise this section whenever you need to refresh your body and energize your mind.

THIS SECTION INCLUDES 13 DYNAMIC SUPER STRETCHES:

LOW dragon LUNGE

This stretch targets your groin area, ankles and hip flexors. It helps to mobilize the pelvis and hips, preparing you for the back bends that follow.

1 Stand with your feet hip-width apart. Move your left foot forwards and place it on the floor in front of you. Rest your right knee and lower leg on the floor behind you. Place your hands lightly on your left knee – right hand on left – to help you balance.

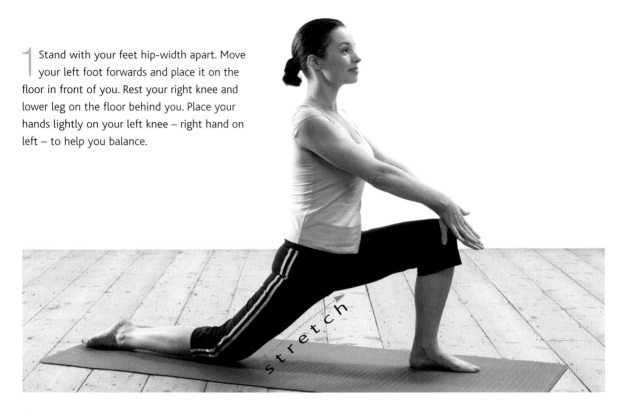

2 Inhale to fill your ribcage and, as you exhale, allow your chest to lower to the inside of your left knee allowing your elbows to rest on the floor level with the arch of your left foot. **Hold for 1–2 minutes.** Return to standing, then repeat on the other side.

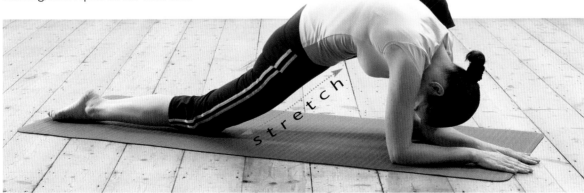

HIGH dragon LUNGE

This version of the Dragon lunge encourages your hips to open more as you rotate your trunk.

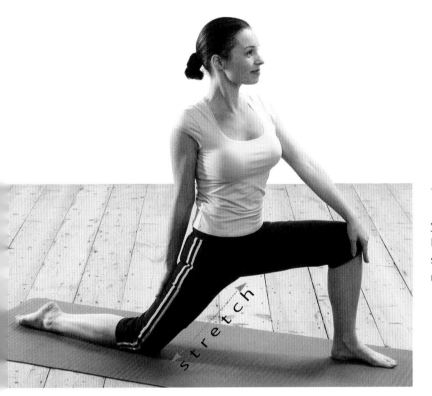

1 From standing position, place your left foot on the floor in front of you. Rest your right knee on the floor behind you. Place your left hand on your left knee and slide your right hand down the back of your right thigh without leaning on your left leg.

2 Inhale to fill your ribcage (without allowing your back to bend) and, as you exhale, slide your right knee away from you. Inhale and, as you exhale, rotate your trunk slightly to the right. **Hold for 1–2 minutes.** Return to standing, then repeat on the other side.

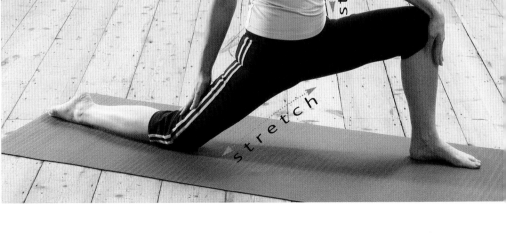

TABLE top STRETCH

A great front shoulder stretch for those with anxiety, general tension or depression. It is also a good stretch if you play racquet sports or have specific upper back or neck tension.

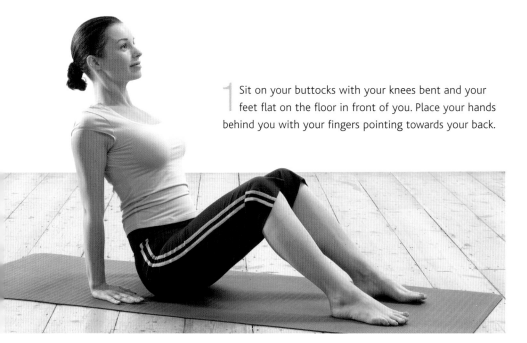

1 Sit on your buttocks with your knees bent and your feet flat on the floor in front of you. Place your hands behind you with your fingers pointing towards your back.

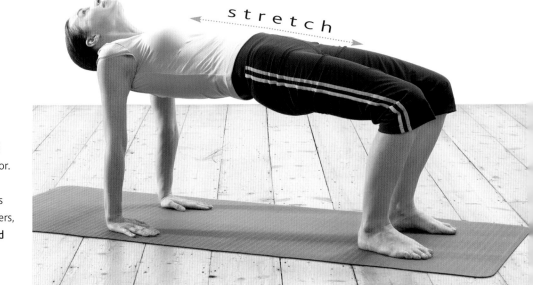

stretch

2 Inhale to fill your ribcage and, as you exhale, lift your hips and lower spine from the floor. Lift as high as you can feeling the stretch across the front of your shoulders, chest and forearms. **Hold for 3–5 breath cycles.**

WIDE forward BEND

A powerful bend that stretches your hamstrings and prepares your groin and hip flexors for further softening and opening. You will also benefit from the inverted blood supply to your face and brain, which improves concentration.

TIP

When in position 2, bend and extend your legs slightly on the inhale breath to release any tension in the back of your knees.

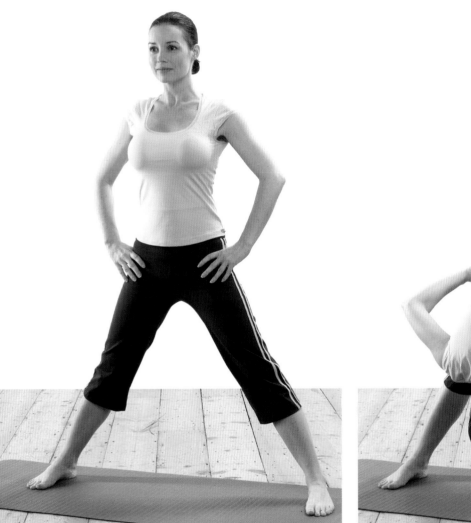

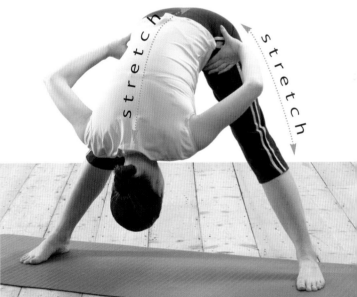

1 Stand with your feet as wide apart as comfortable and place your hands on your hips. Inhale to fill your ribcage, press your hands into your hip bones to lift and broaden your upper trunk.

2 Inhale and,, as you exhale, hinge forwards at your hips. Continue to lower your trunk slowly towards the floor, while keeping the length in your spine. **Hold for 5–8 breath cycles.**

STANDING squat

This squat stretch opens and strengthens the large IT band tendon found in your thighs. It also increases your body temperature, helping your muscles to relax further.

TIP

You can broaden the ball of your left foot to help you balance.

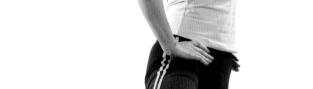

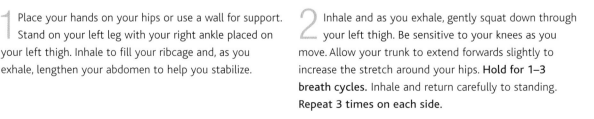

stretch

1 Place your hands on your hips or use a wall for support. Stand on your left leg with your right ankle placed on your left thigh. Inhale to fill your ribcage and, as you exhale, lengthen your abdomen to help you stabilize.

2 Inhale and as you exhale, gently squat down through your left thigh. Be sensitive to your knees as you move. Allow your trunk to extend forwards slightly to increase the stretch around your hips. **Hold for 1–3 breath cycles.** Inhale and return carefully to standing. **Repeat 3 times on each side.**

VARIATION

If you find it difficult to balance in this position, you can do this stretch sitting down with one leg outstretched and the foot of the other leg resting on your thigh as you hinge forwards.

THIGH stretch

This lengthens the four quadriceps muscles that travel up the front of your thighs. Stretching these large muscles helps to release knee tension and improves your posture by working the muscles that connect to your hips.

1 Stand with your feet hip-width apart. Bend your left knee slightly and bring your right ankle to your right buttock. Inhale and take hold of your ankle. Place your left hand on your left hip to help you balance. Exhale and lengthen through your tailbone to deepen the stretch. **Hold the stretch for 5–8 breath cycles**, then repeat on the other side.

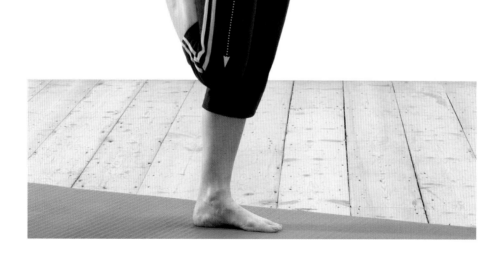

STANDING hamstring STRETCH

A useful stretch that you can do throughout the day; you can do it anywhere and you don't have to warm up. It lengthens your hamstrings, which can become tired from sitting all day, and releases tension from your lower spine.

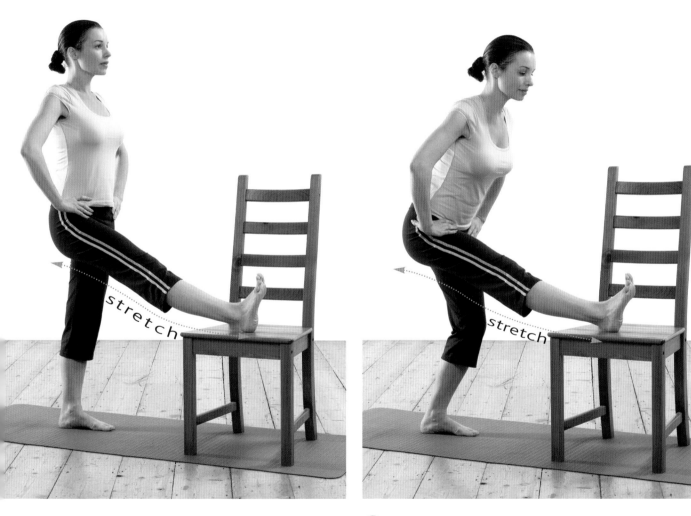

1 Stand opposite a chair or step with your hands on your hips. Bend your left knee slightly and place your right foot on the chair or step, foot flexed.

2 Inhale and lengthen your spine. Keeping your hands on your hips, lengthen through your right leg. Drawing your thigh muscles to the bone, extend your trunk forwards to deepen the stretch along the back of your right leg. **Hold for 5–8 breath cycles**, then repeat on the other side.

RUNNER'S lunge

Familiar to runners and other sportspeople, this is a great stretch for lengthening your leg muscles and opening your hip joints. It also helps to maintain body temperature, making it easier to elongate your muscles.

1 Stand in a wide stance with your right leg forward and your left leg back. Slowly bend your right leg to a 90° angle and raise your left heel off the floor. Inhale and, as you exhale, straighten your back leg. As you inhale and exhale again, deepen into the front lunge, pushing into the ball of your left foot.

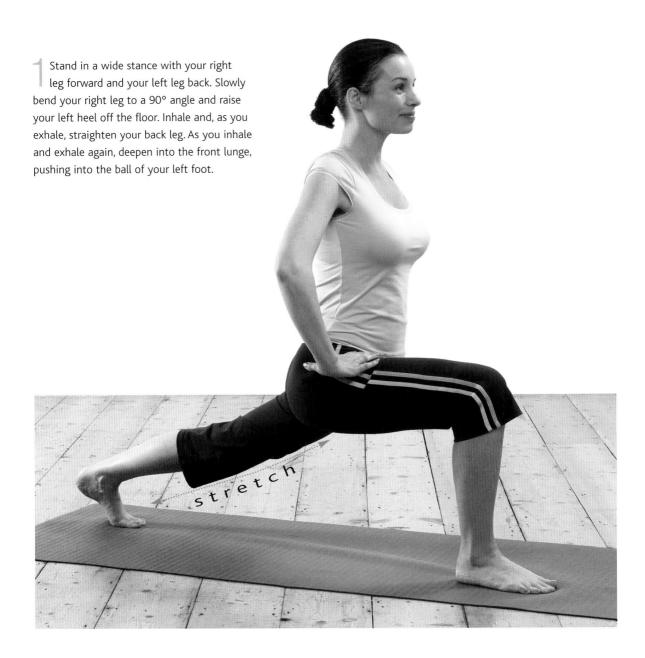

stretch

2 Inhale to fill your ribcage and raise your left arm in front and your right arm behind you. Rotate your trunk to the right. **Hold for 5 breath cycles**, then repeat on the other side.

stretch

stretch

stretch

KNEELING side STRETCH

This stretch helps to lengthen the sides of your waist and
soften the muscles that support your lumbar (lower) spine.
It also provides a slight rotation of the trunk muscles from
the pelvis that helps to soften the hips.

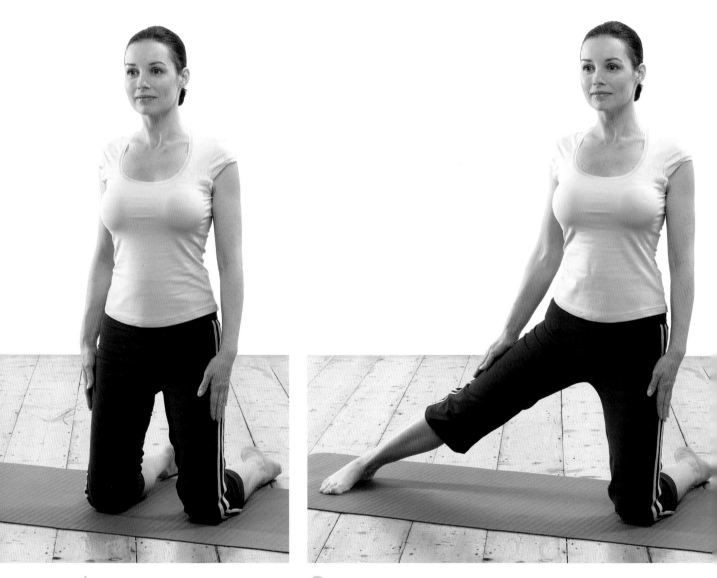

1 Kneel with your knees hip-width
apart and your spine long. Exhale
to empty your abdomen.

2 Inhale and extend your right leg out to your right
side. Keep your right foot central and grounded.
Exhale and lengthen your abdomen to help you stabilize.

s t r e t c h

3 Inhale and raise your left arm up and, as you exhale, slide your right arm down your right leg. Extend your left arm over your head, stretching your waist and upper back. **Hold for 5 breath cycles,** then repeat on the other side.

SEATED forward BEND

An effective stretch that helps to lengthen your hamstrings, which in turn releases tension from the lower back. This is a great exercise to help you get moving in the morning.

TIP

If you can feel your shoulders lifting towards your ears during this forward bend, relax your arms and do not hold your legs.

1 Sit on the floor with your legs stretched in front of you and your feet flexed. Have your ankles, knees and thighs together and your hands resting on the floor beside your hips. Draw your thigh muscles into your thigh bones. Inhale and lengthen your spine.

2 Exhale as you extend your trunk towards your legs, without dropping your head or chest. Inhale and, as you exhale, extend towards your legs again. Rest your arms gently on either your shins or feet, but do not pull through your arms. **Hold for 1–2 breath cycles, then release slowly.**

stretch

stretch

SEATED hamstring STRETCH

This stretch targets the hamstrings connection to your spine, helping both to elongate. This helps to improve flexibility and alleviate lower back pain.

1 Sit on the floor, legs stretched in front of you and your spine tall. Bring your left foot towards your right buttock bone, then bring your right foot as close to your left shin as possible. Keep your right foot grounded.

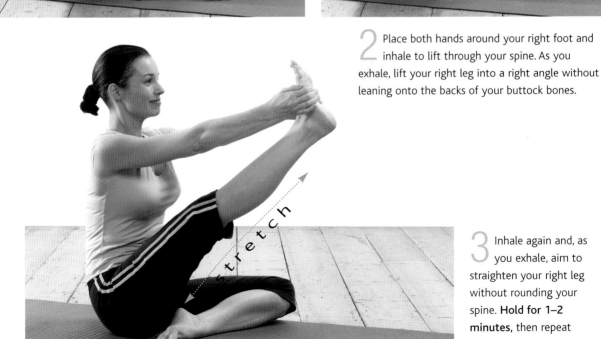

2 Place both hands around your right foot and inhale to lift through your spine. As you exhale, lift your right leg into a right angle without leaning onto the backs of your buttock bones.

3 Inhale again and, as you exhale, aim to straighten your right leg without rounding your spine. **Hold for 1–2 minutes,** then repeat on the other side.

OUTER hamstring STRETCH

This version of the Seated hamstring stretch requires greater flexibility and good balance. It also targets your inner thighs, groin muscles and the muscles that connect to your lower spine.

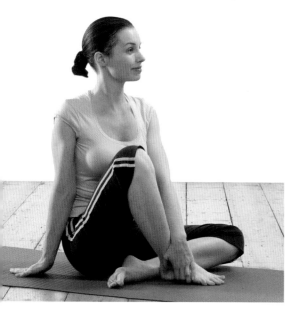

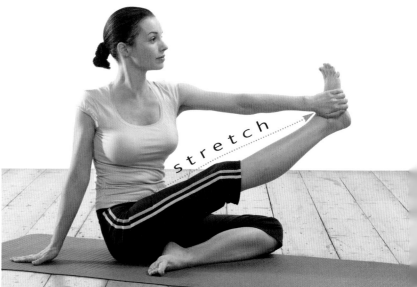

1 Sit on the floor with your legs stretched in front of you. Bring your left foot towards your right buttock bone. Bring your right foot to your left shin. Place your left hand around your right foot and sit tall.

2 Inhale and as you exhale, lift and extend your right leg and take it across the mid-line of your body to your left.

3 Inhale and extend your right arm behind you keeping your spine long. Exhale and lengthen your abdomen to help stretch your inner thigh. **Hold for 1–2 minutes**, then repeat on the other side.

INNER hamstring STRETCH

This variation of the Seated hamstring stretch lengthens the
IT band tendon located in the outer edge of your thighs.

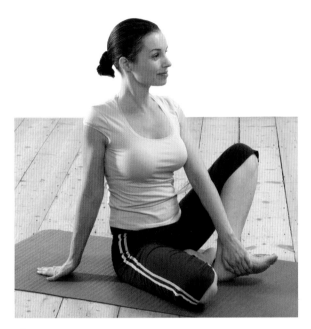

1 Sit on the floor with your legs stretched in front of
you. Bring your right foot towards your left buttock
bone. Bring your left foot to your right shin. Place your
left hand around the inside of your left foot and sit tall.

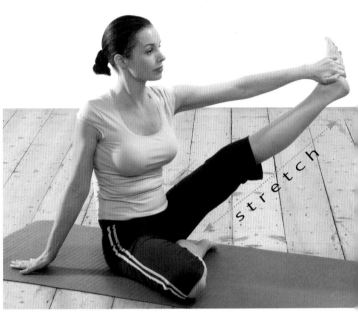

2 Inhale and, as you exhale, lift your left leg forwards
towards the mid-line of your body, then take it out
to your left side.

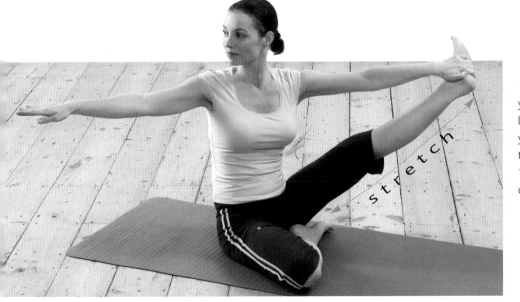

3 Inhale and extend
your right arm to
your right side maintaining
length in your spine. Move
your gaze so you look over
the right shoulder. **Hold for
1–2 minutes,** then repeat
on the other side.

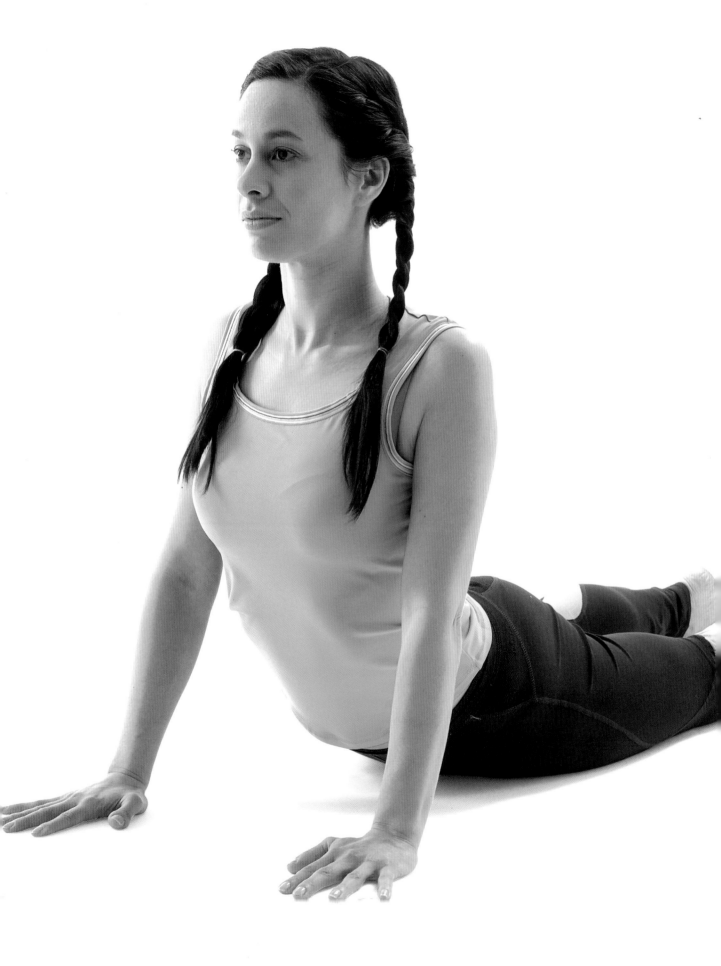

STRETCHING YOUR SPINE

When it comes to movement, the spine is the most important part of your body. It forms the central axis, which houses your nervous system. Therefore, any tension that builds up over time in and around the spine will affect your ability to function to your full potential.

Lots of sitting around, too much of one type of activity and lack of strength in your abdomen will soon distort the neutral shape of your spine. This can produce problems with movement and can cause pain and discomfort.

The stretches in this section help to prevent back pain and to maintain suppleness within your spine. Some of these techniques need to be undertaken with care and attention as rushing or jarring a movement could lead to injury. Take your time to move in and out of the stretches. You can spend a little longer on this section and it is advised you do this section every other day.

THIS SECTION INCLUDES 9 SPINE SUPER STRETCHES:

CURVED roll DOWN

An effective exercise that stretches and relaxes your spine and neck. It also helps to strengthen your core back and abdominal muscles, which can help tone and strengthen your abdominal area.

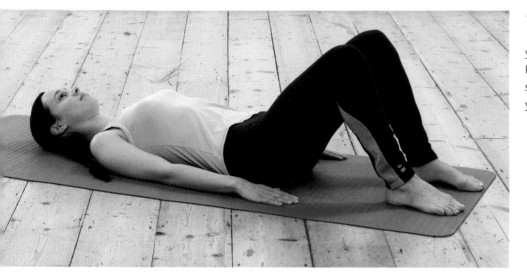

1 Lie on your back with your knees bent and your feet flat on the floor. Place your arms by the sides of your body with your palms facing down.

2 Inhale to fill your ribcage and, as you exhale, lift your lower body from the floor to bring your knees towards your forehead. Rest your knees on your forehead. **Hold for 1–3 minutes.**

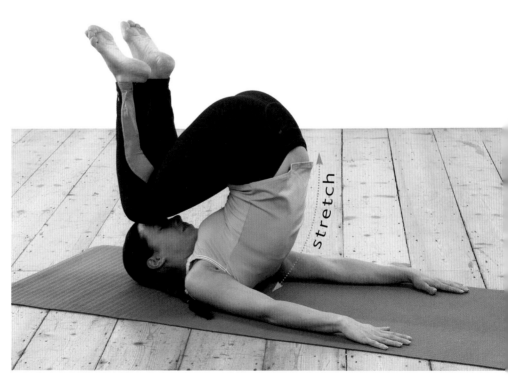

stretch

TIP

Try to keep your shoulders
as relaxed as possible and use
your abdominal muscles
to roll down without
holding your breath.

3 Inhale and, as you exhale, roll down your
spine slowly to return your feet to the floor.
Use your core abdominal muscles to control the
movement and to stop your feet dropping to
the floor. **Repeat 5 times.**

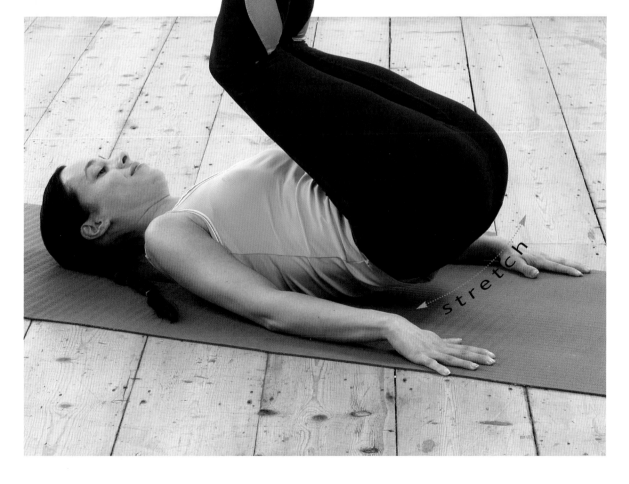

stretch

FOLDED pose

This technique provides a gentle stretch for your spine and helps to loosen your hip joints.

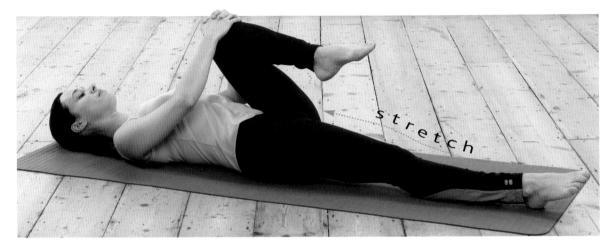

1 Lie on your back with your legs stretched along the floor. Inhale and draw your left knee in towards your chest. Place both hands around your raised knee. Exhale and lengthen your abdominals, keeping your spine in a neutral position, without your spine arching or rounding as you move. **Hold for 3 breath cycles.** Inhale to fill your ribcage and, as you exhale, return your leg to the floor. **Repeat on alternate sides up to 5 times on each side.**

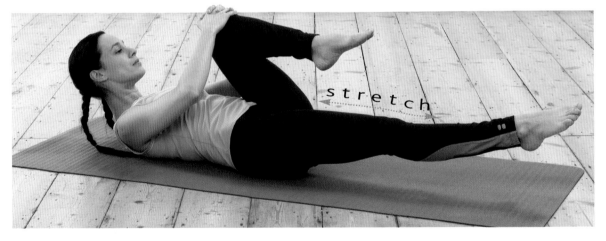

VARIATION

For a deeper stretch inhale and bring your forehead towards your knee and raise your extended leg slightly off the floor. Exhale and curl back down slowly to the floor.

SPINE twist

This technique helps to release tension in several muscles, including your lower back, abdominals and hips. It also helps to stimulate your energy channels that your breath and energy run through, helping to nourish the immune, glandular and thyroid systems.

1 Lie on your back with your legs stretched along the floor and your arms out to your sides level with your shoulders. Inhale and, as you exhale, bring your right leg into your chest, followed by your left leg. Inhale and cross your left leg over your right leg and lock your foot around your ankle. Exhale and lengthen your abdomen, while keeping your shoulders broad.

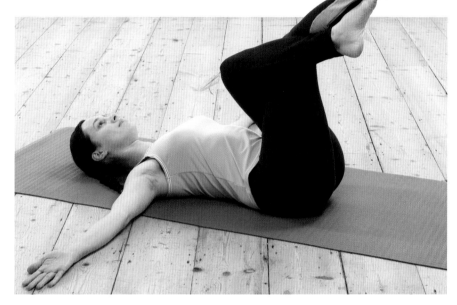

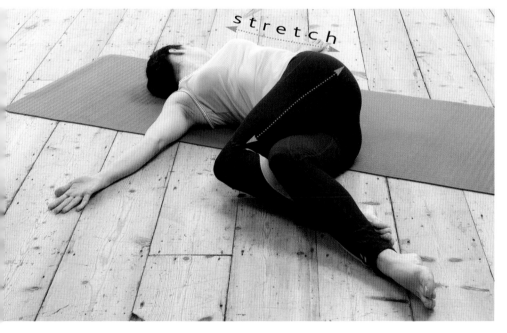

2 Inhale and, as you exhale, rotate your trunk and lower both legs to the right to the floor. Turn your head to the left. **Hold for 1 minute, breathing deeply,** then repeat on the other side.

VARIATION

To increase the stretch, place your hand on your knees to hold them closer to the floor. Also, aim to draw your knees higher towards your shoulders to vary the stretch.

SNAIL stretch

The Snail stretch stretches the entire spinal column and is a very pleasant stretch to be done slowly. Each stage of this stretch increases in movement and intensity, so progress at your own level.

CAUTION
If you have any back problems, approach this sequence with care.

TIP
Keep the back of your shoulders broad on the floor so that your neck does not press into the floor. If your knees do not touch your forehead do not force them; in time they will lower as your back softens.

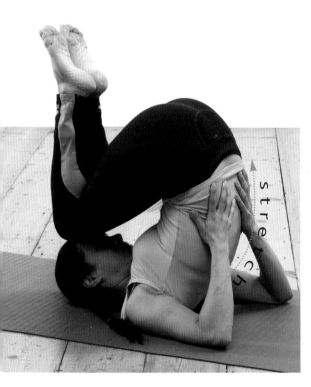

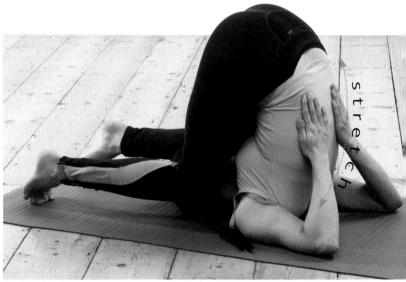

1 Lie on your back with your knees bent and feet resting on the floor. Place your arms on the floor with your palms pressing down. Inhale and roll your legs up to bring your knees to your forehead. Exhale and lengthen and empty your abdomen. Place your hands on your lower back for support. **Hold for 1–3 minutes.**

2 Inhale and extend your legs over your head and place the balls of your feet on the floor. Exhale and relax your legs allowing your knees to drop towards your ears. Keep your hands on your lower back for support. **Hold for 1–3 minutes, breathing steadily.**

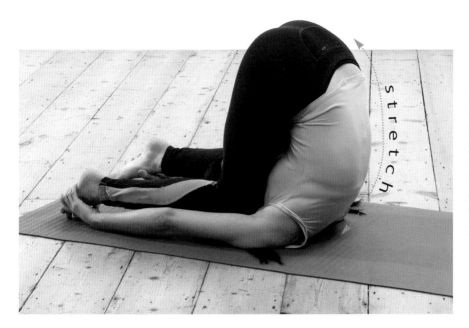

3 Inhale and, as you exhale, take your right arm to hold the sole of your right foot. Inhale and, as you exhale, take your left arm to hold the sole of your left foot. Relax your shoulders into the floor. Keep your hips low and your legs bent. **Hold for 1 minute.**

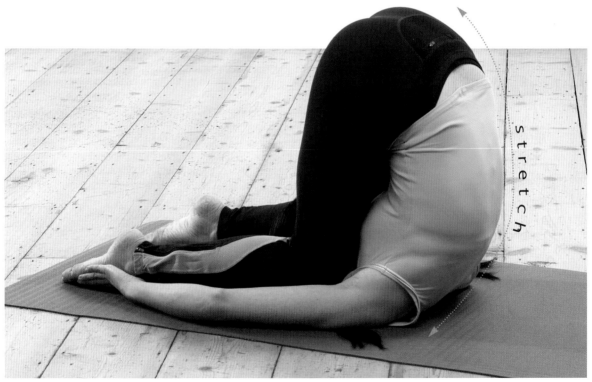

4 Inhale and as you exhale, bend your knees back to the floor. Inhale and, as you exhale, lengthen the front of your ankles to release your ankle joints. Your feet will be flat on the floor. Keep the back of your shoulders broad. **Hold for 1 minute**, then return to original position.

VARIATION

If your feet do not touch the floor behind your head, place your feet on a cushion or the edge of a sofa.

the SEAL

A great counterbalance to the Snail stretch, the Seal is a back bend that releases stiffness in your lower spine. It also helps to re-establish the natural lumbar curve of the lower spine that is often lost when we sit for a long time.

TIP

Use your arms to lift your ribcage. As you lift up try to maintain a feeling of softness in your back.

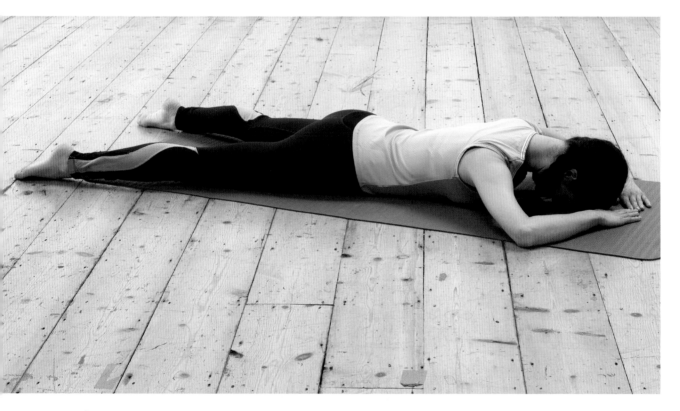

1 Lie on your stomach with your legs long about 1¹/₂ shoulder-widths apart. Place your hands in a diamond shape in front of your head with your elbows out to the side. Inhale to fill your ribcage and extend your ribcage forwards and up from the floor. Exhale and **hold for 30 seconds breathing comfortably.**

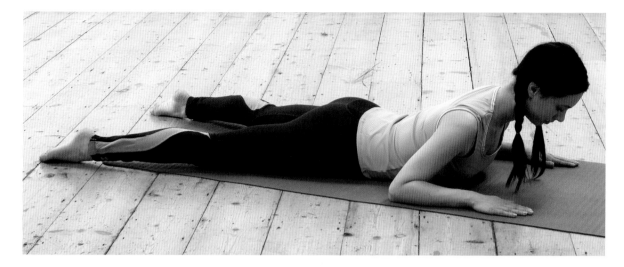

2 Bring your elbows in towards your ribcage. Inhale
 to fill your lungs and, as you exhale, lift your ribcage
forwards and up, resting slightly on your elbows. Inhale
and, as you exhale, feel the connection of your stomach
muscles to your spine. **Hold for 1 minute.**

stretch

3 Drop back down to the floor and extend your hands
 in front of your shoulders, keeping your shoulders
back towards your hips. Inhale to fill your ribcage and, as
you exhale, lift forwards and up onto your hands, with
your hips still in contact with the floor. **Hold for 1 minute.**

the SADDLE

This stretches your feet, knees and thighs. It also arches your lumbar spine and sacral vertebrae (found in your lower spine) that can become tight through long bouts of sitting or inactivity. Each stage increases the stretch.

TIP

Coming out of the Saddle can be tricky, so roll or lean onto your side and unfold your legs one by one.

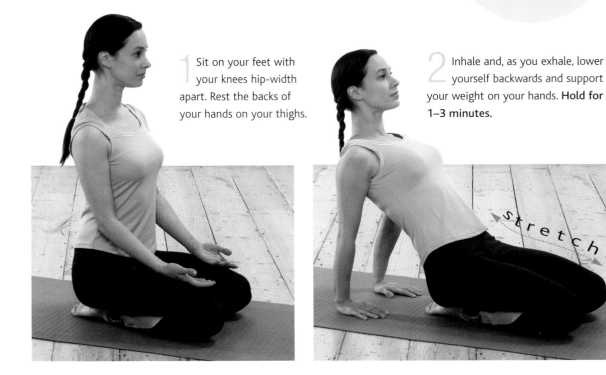

1 Sit on your feet with your knees hip-width apart. Rest the backs of your hands on your thighs.

2 Inhale and, as you exhale, lower yourself backwards and support your weight on your hands. **Hold for 1–3 minutes.**

stretch

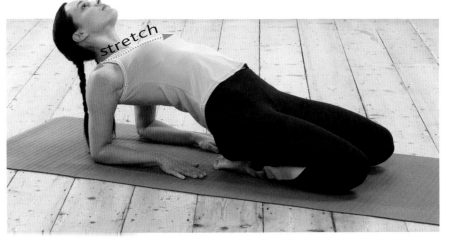

stretch

3 If the stretch feels easy, move on to your elbows. **Hold for 1–3 minutes.**

VARIATION

To progress further with this exercise, arch your spine slightly and inhale. As you exhale, slide your spine downwards towards the floor and relax your arms by the side of your body. **Hold for 1–3 minutes.**

TRIPOD stretch

A strong stretch that strengthens your upper body and works all the muscles in your torso. It is also a nice counter-pose to the earlier forward bends and prepares your body for more back bends.

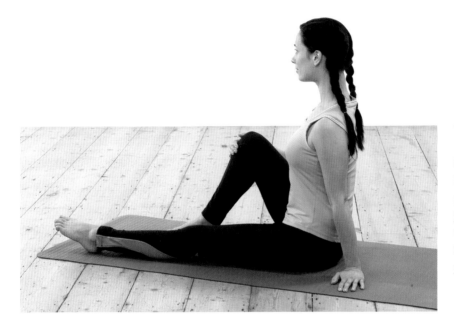

1 Sit with your spine tall and your legs stretched out in front of you. Place your right hand onto your right knee, and place your left hand behind you on the floor. Bend your right knee and place your right foot level with the inside of your left knee.

2 Push your pelvis up as high as possible, using your left arm and upper back. At the same time sweep your right arm in a circular motion across your body into an extended position to your right side. Turn to the left to look at the floor while stretching your right arm over your head, then look towards your right hand. **Hold for 3–5 breath cycles,** then repeat on the other side. **Repeat 2–3 times.**

SNAIL walk

A great stretch for relaxing and working the muscles in your spine. You can feel the benefit from the base of your head down to your tailbone.

TIP

You will find that you will slow down as you feel the deepening of the stretch run more intensely through your spine. Take plenty of time to hold this stretch for a few breath cycles before moving over to the other side.

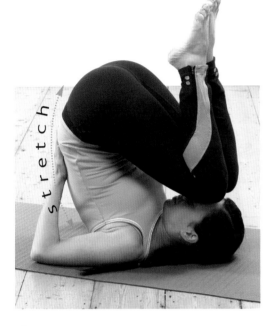

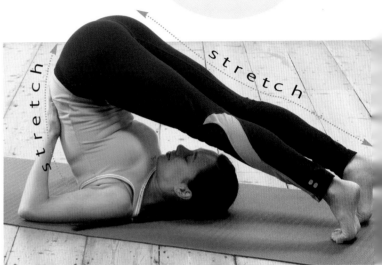

1 Lie on your back with your knees bent in towards your chest. Inhale and, as you exhale, roll your knees up towards your forehead. Support your lower back with your hands.

2 Inhale and, as you exhale, extend your feet over your head so the balls of your feet are grounded on the floor hip-width apart. Rest your hands on your lower back with your fingers pointing towards the ceiling.

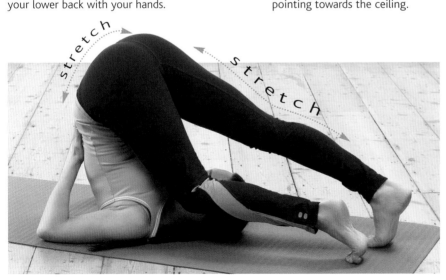

3 Inhale and, as you exhale, bend your left leg while extending your right leg. Allow your pelvis to tilt to the left. **Hold for 3 breath cycles.** Inhale and exhale as you return both feet to centre, then repeat on the other side. **Repeat 15 times.**

COBRA rib OPENER

This stretch encourages space in your intestines and helps to aid digestion. It also strengthens the natural lumbar curve of your spine, which can be lost through bending forwards and sitting for long periods of time.

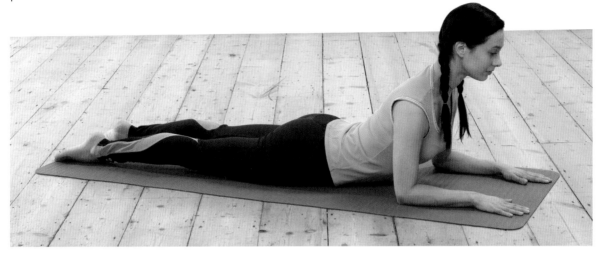

1 Lie on your front and bring your elbows in towards your ribcage. Inhale and, as you exhale, gently lift your ribcage forwards and up.

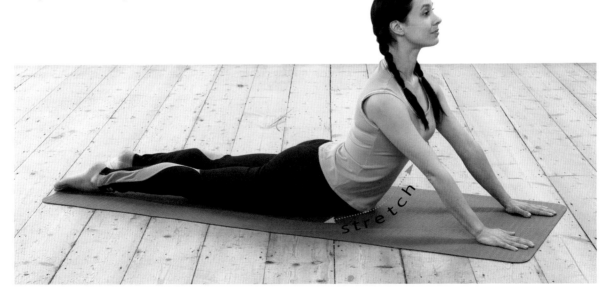

stretch

2 Inhale and, as you exhale, slide up onto your hands. Keep your shoulder blades away from your ears.
Hold for 1–2 minutes, breathing naturally.

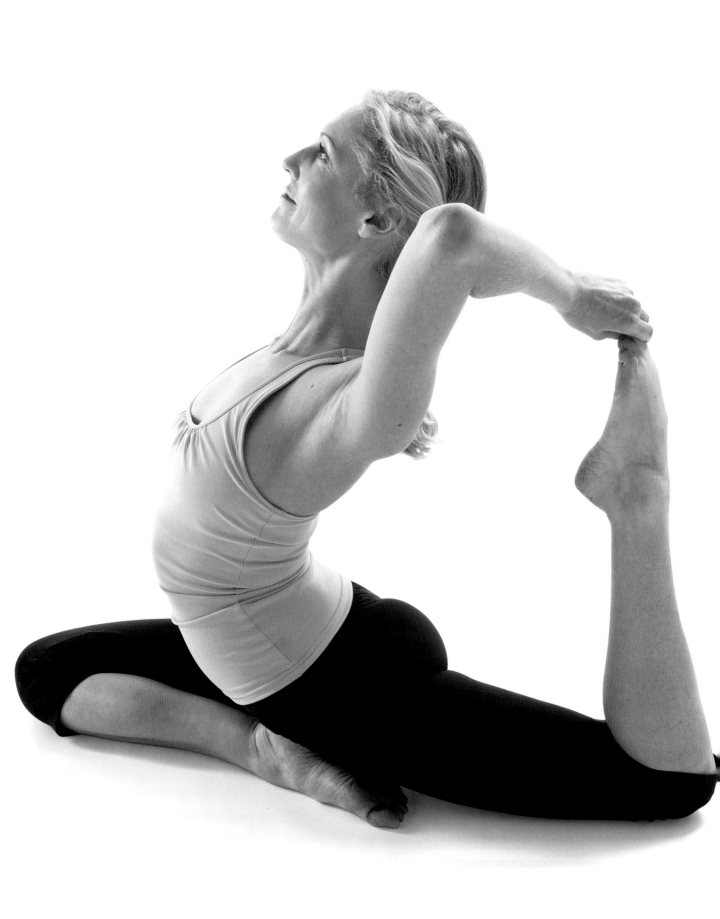

STRETCHING YOUR HIPS AND LEGS

These stretches focus on your hips and legs, areas of the body where most tension builds up. Due to the long hours most of us spend sitting, it is very common for the hamstring muscles in the back of the legs to become very tight, and because we don't tend to use the full range of movement through our hip sockets, our hips also become locked and stiff.

Stiff hips feel very uncomfortable, but over time we can get used to these sensations and they become 'normal'. It is important to practise the stretches in this section to familiarize yourself with the range of movement and flexibility in your legs and hips. Some of the stretches may be uncomfortable at first, but continue to practise until they become more comfortable and familiar.

THIS SECTION INCLUDES 12 HIP AND LEG SUPER STRETCHES:

SLEEPING swan

This stretch rotates your legs to stretch the muscles and connective tissues in the outside of your buttocks and thighs. It also stretches your hip flexors.

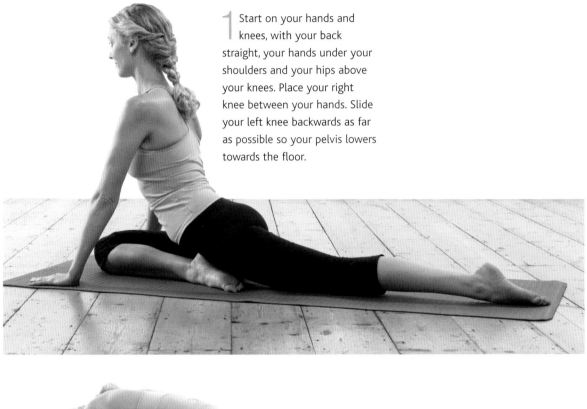

1 Start on your hands and knees, with your back straight, your hands under your shoulders and your hips above your knees. Place your right knee between your hands. Slide your left knee backwards as far as possible so your pelvis lowers towards the floor.

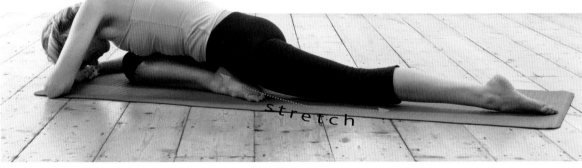

2 Lean forwards and take some of your weight onto your elbows. Tuck your right foot into your groin – your pelvis should be suspended just above the floor with tension in your hip and thigh. **Hold for 1–3 minutes**, then repeat on the other side.

VARIATION

As you become more flexible try this more challenging option. Move your front foot further forwards and try to rest your chest on your leg.

UPRIGHT swan

This version of the Swan stretch adds a back-bend movement; this helps to stretch your back leg hip flexors more deeply.

TIP

When raising your back leg, keep your pelvis down and try not to let it twist as you move.

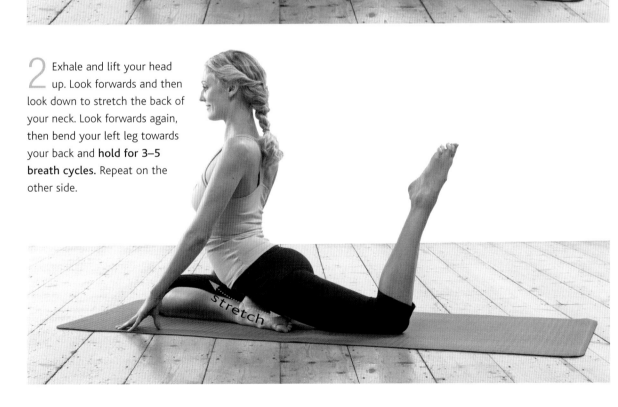

1 Start on your hands and knees, with your back straight, your hands under your shoulders and your hips above your knees. Place your right knee between your hands. Slide your left knee backwards as far as possible so your pelvis lowers towards the floor.

2 Exhale and lift your head up. Look forwards and then look down to stretch the back of your neck. Look forwards again, then bend your left leg towards your back and **hold for 3–5 breath cycles.** Repeat on the other side.

stretch

FOLDED splits

This stretch really makes your body feel good. It targets your inner groin area and lumbar spine and opens your back muscles. It also helps to tone your waist and legs.

1 Sit with your legs stretched out on the floor in a straddle position. Your sitting bones should be grounded and your spine tall and long. Inhale and lengthen your abdomen to sit up straight.

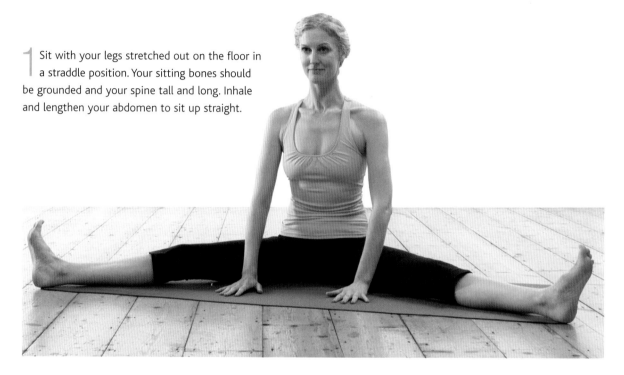

2 Exhale and as you do so allow your chest to lower towards the floor. Keep your spine long and your chest open. Keep the backs of your knees as close to the floor as possible. **Hold for 1–2 minutes, breathing evenly.**

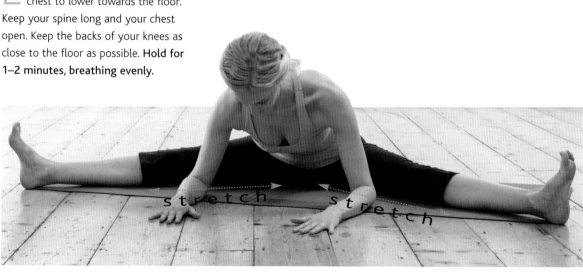

stretch   stretch

SEATED side STRETCH

This is similar to the Folded splits, but this variation also softens your inner hip joints and the sides of your back.

1 Sit with your legs stretched out in a straddle position. Your sitting bones should be grounded, your spine long and your abdomen lengthened. Inhale and, as you exhale, bend to your left, reaching along the inside of your left leg with your left arm. Exhale and **hold for 1 minute.**

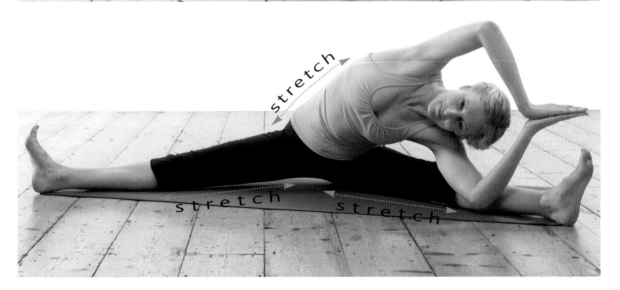

2 Inhale and extend your right arm upwards in line with your right shoulder. Exhale and stretch your right arm over in line with your ear. Aim to bring your hands together. Exhale and **hold for 1–3 minutes,** then repeat on the other side.

VARIATION
If you are very flexible, aim to hold the ball of your foot. However, this may not be where you feel the stretch the most, so adjust your position to suit your body and where you feel the most obvious stretch sensation that can be held without aggression.

FROG stretch

A dynamic stretch to target your inner hip sockets and groin area, the Frog stretch helps to relieve hard-working muscles that can become tight over time. You can relax into this stretch allowing gravity to do most of the work.

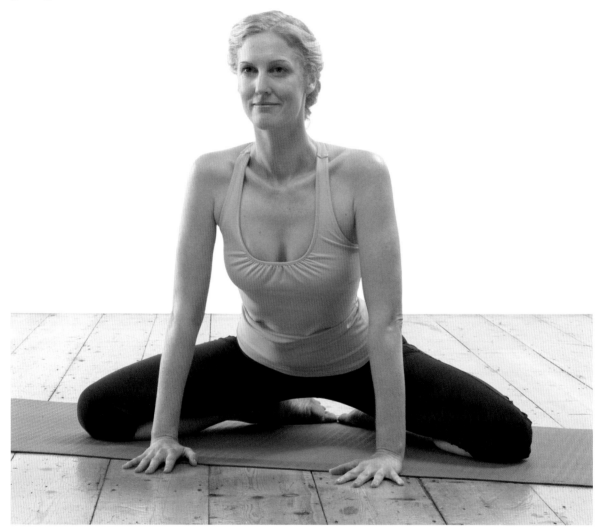

1 Start in a crouching position with your hands flat on the floor. Take your knees as wide as they will go and with the tips of your big toes together. Inhale to fill your ribcage and, as you exhale, press your sitting bones back towards your heels. Place your hands on the floor in front of you with your palms down. Lean forwards until you feel tension. **Hold for 1–3 minutes.**

VARIATION

An easy option is to sit with your back tall and the soles of your feet together. Inhale and place your hands on the inside of your calf muscles. As you exhale, ease your knees away from each other gently to increase the stretch.

HALF saddle STRETCH

This is a variation of the full Saddle (see page 64). This version is done with one leg at a time and encourages the correct position of the lumbar spine. It also stretches the front of your thighs.

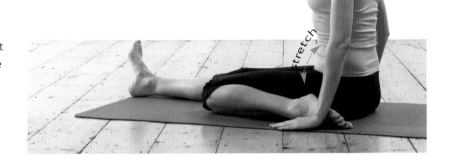

1 Sit upright with your left foot tucked backwards by the side of your left buttock bone. Rest your hands on the floor. Inhale to fill your ribcage and, as you exhale, allow gravity to stretch the front of your left hip.

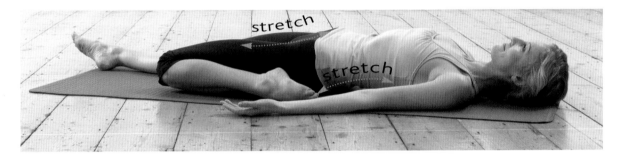

2 Inhale to fill your ribcage and, as you exhale, allow your spine to extend backwards and rest on your elbows. Release back onto your back. Relax in this position and breathe freely **holding for 1–3 minutes.** Repeat on the other side.

VARIATIONS

If your left knee lifts off the floor you can stay on step 1 to soften the thigh muscles first before you progress further. If the stretch is too intense, bend your right leg so your right foot is flat on the floor to alleviate any stress in the spine.

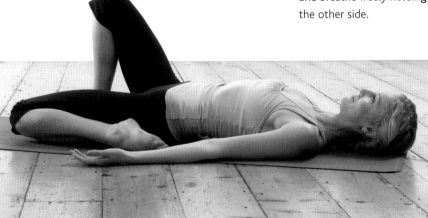

PASSIVE butterfly

Your inner hip joints can become stiff from too little movement or from sitting for long periods of time. If you find this stretch painful, your hips have become tight; aim to do this stretch little and often to ease them.

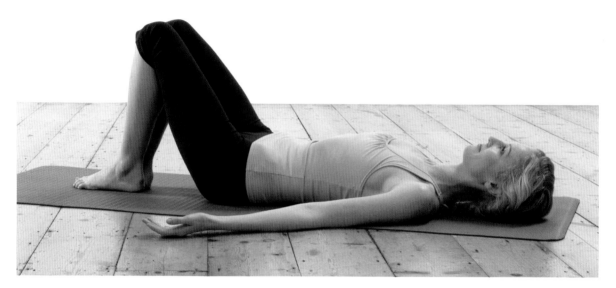

1 Lie on your back with your legs bent and your feet flat on the floor. Your ankles, knees and thighs should touch. Rest your arms by the sides of your body with your palms turned upwards.

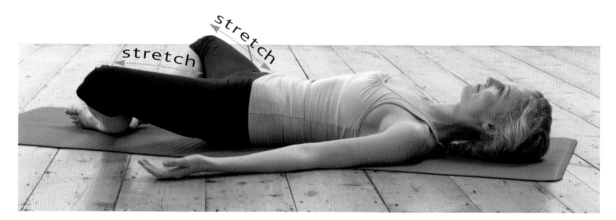

2 Inhale to fill your ribcage and, as you exhale, allow your knees to float apart bringing the soles of your feet together. Rest here and let gravity relax your hips and back. **Hold for 1–5 minutes.**

DEEP outer hip RELEASE

A reverse movement to the Passive butterfly, this stretch provides immediate relief from any discomfort you may feel now. It also opens the muscles running along your outer hip sockets, maximizing more movement around your hip joints and legs.

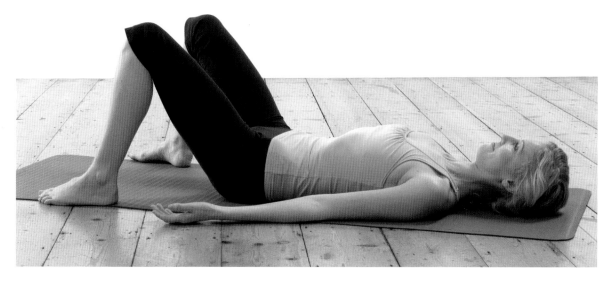

1 Lie on your back with your knees bent and your feet flat on the floor. Place your feet as wide apart as possible, while still keeping them in parallel. Keep your spine long and your abdomen lengthened.

2 Inhale and, as you exhale, allow your knees to drop in towards each other. Rest your knees gently together and allow gravity to soften the outer hip sockets. To deepen the stretch, move your feet a little further away from each other. **Rest in this position for 1–5 minutes.**

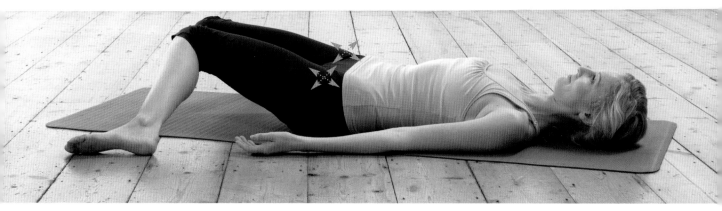

HURDLE stretch

This stretch reverses the Butterfly stretch again and changes the angle on your back hip so you stretch through your lumbar spine as well as your groin.

TIP

Try to keep your ribcage lifted and your back long. It is very easy to round your spine and collapse the chest, which restricts breathing and misaligns the spine posture.

1 Sit with your legs in front of you with your back tall and long. Take your left leg behind you so your knee is in line with your hip.

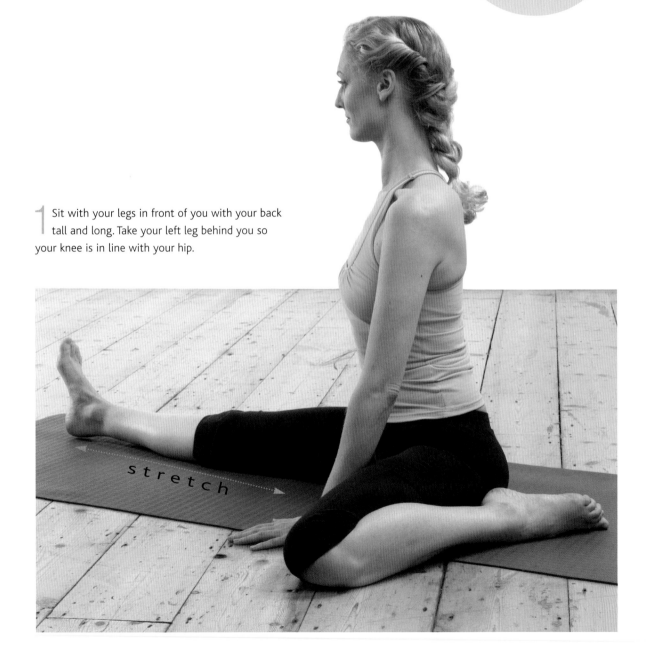

stretch

2 Inhale and lengthen your spine. As you exhale, allow your trunk to extend over your right leg. Inhale to fill your ribcage. As you exhale, draw your abdomen in towards your spine. **Hold for 2–3 minutes, using your breath to help you stretch further.** Repeat on the other side.

stretch

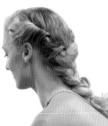

VARIATION

If you have any problems with your knees, extend your left leg out to the side so your leg is straight and your knee joint relaxed.

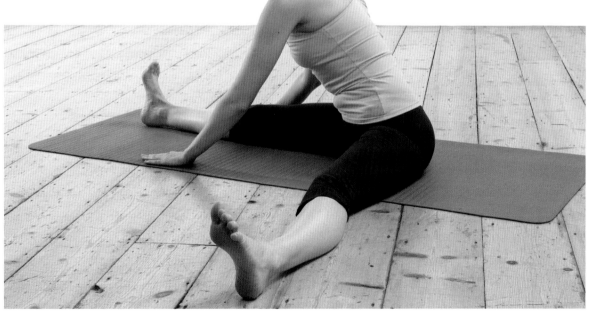

SPLITS hip OPENER

This exercise stretches your groin, ankles and hip flexors. It encourages the pelvis to be free in its movements, bringing more mobility into your lumbar spine and strength into your abdominals. There are three stages to this stretch.

TIP

Check that your back stays upright and your pelvis does not push forwards. Draw your abdominals in towards your spine to help you stabilize.

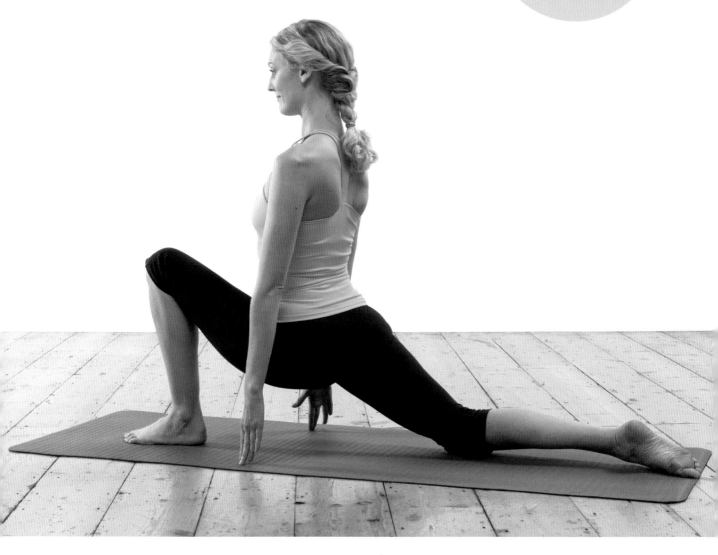

1 Start by kneeling on the floor. Place your left foot forwards and extend your right leg behind you. Place both hands on the floor or on your front knee for support. Inhale to fill your lungs and, as you exhale, press your hips forwards. **Hold for 1–2 minutes.**

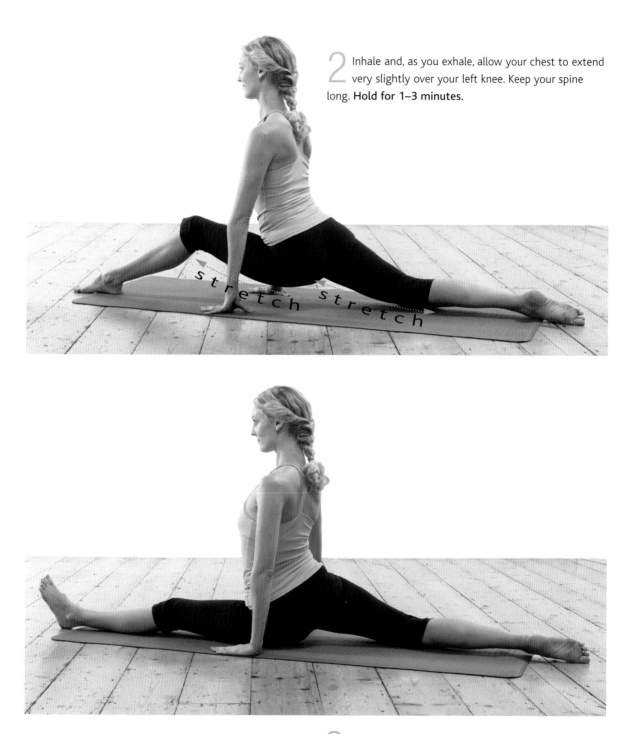

2 Inhale and, as you exhale, allow your chest to extend very slightly over your left knee. Keep your spine long. **Hold for 1–3 minutes.**

stretch stretch

3 Inhale and, as you exhale, slide your back leg away behind you bringing your groin towards the floor. **Breathe naturally and hold for 1–3 minutes.**

INSIDE hip OPENER

Another joint softener for your knees, hips and ankles. It also promotes flexibility around your internal hip joint muscles.

TIP

Try to keep your pelvis in contact with the floor at all times. If it starts to lift, exhale and try to draw it back towards the floor.

1 Lie on your back and tuck your right foot in towards your groin. Inhale and bring your left foot to the top of your right thigh.

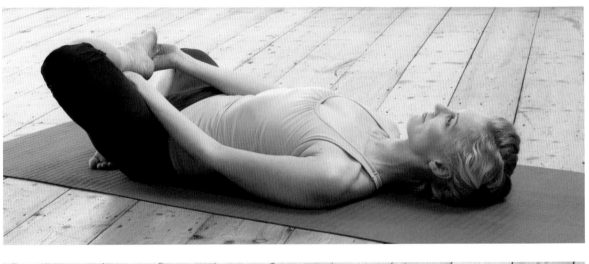

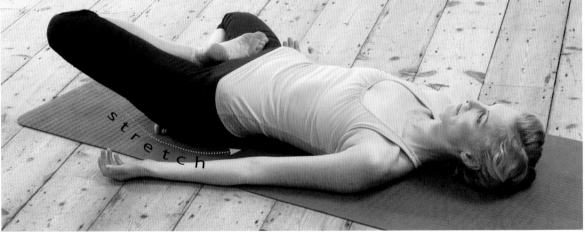

stretch

2 Inhale to fill your ribcage and, as you exhale, let your left leg relax on your inner thigh, allowing gravity to help soften the hip. Exhale and relax with your hands by the sides of your body. **Hold for 1–3 minutes.** Repeat on the other side.

VARIATION

To deepen this stretch as your flexibility improves, move your left foot further into the inner thigh of the opposite leg, deepening the opening around your hip.

OUTSIDE hip OPENER

This is a reverse to the previous stretches, targeting your outer hip flexors. These flexors can become tight and stiff, which can lead to tightening and pain in the lower back muscles.

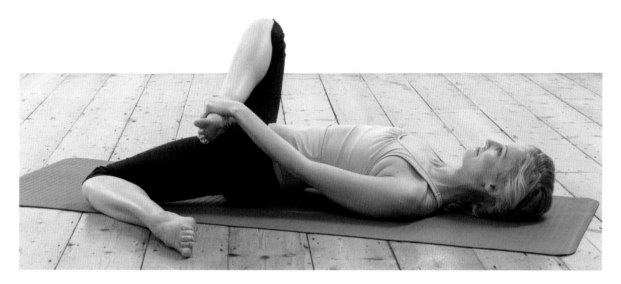

1 Lie on your back and drop your left knee inwards towards the floor. Bring your left foot up towards your bottom. Place your right foot on the top of your left thigh.

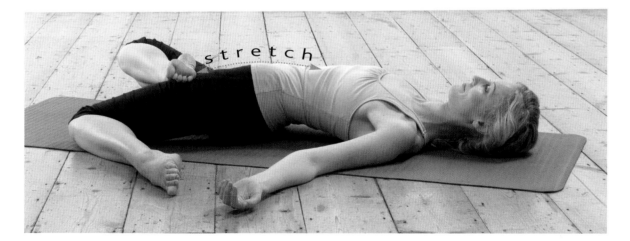

stretch

2 Inhale to fill your ribcage and, as you exhale, allow gravity and the weight of your right leg to soften the left hip joint and your right leg to drop towards the floor. **Hold for 1–3 minutes.** Repeat on the other side.

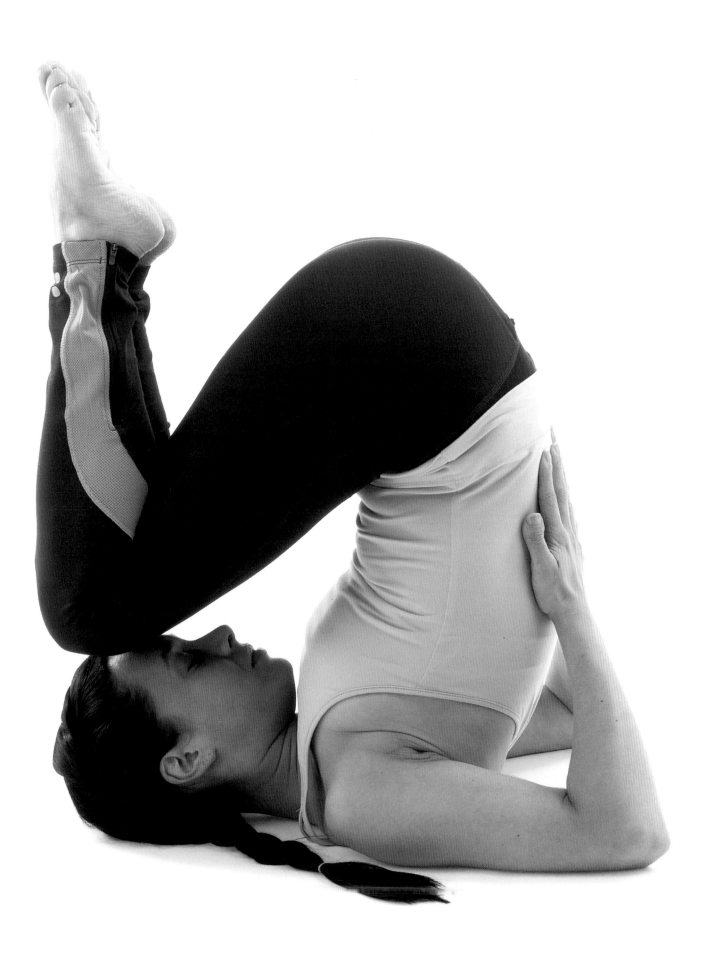

STRETCHING YOUR HIPS, LEGS AND SPINE

This section follows on from the work of the previous chapter with more challenging exercises, designed to challenge your spine as well. The hips, legs and spine are key movement points for the body, so it is important to stretch regularly to release tension in these areas. Unrelieved, chronic tension can also affect your nervous system.

If you have only done *Stretching your hips and legs* once or twice and find the stretches challenging, then skip this section completely. When you find the stretches straightforward, continue with this section or replace some of the exercises for variety.

As you move deeper into your body you will spend longer in the stretches. This is a sign that things are getting easier and you should go with the flow and enjoy getting to know your body on a more intimate level.

THIS SECTION INCLUDES 11 HIP, LEG AND SPINE SUPER STRETCHES:

- Square stretch (see pages 86–7)
- Spine stimulation (see page 88)
- Spine arch (see page 89)
- Easy back stretch (see page 90)
- Spine twist (see page 91)
- Cross-leg forward bend (see page 92)
- Supine leg stretch (see page 93)
- Supine thigh stretch (see page 94)
- Supine groin stretch (see page 95)
- Rocking stretch (see page 96)
- Wide plough stretch (see page 97)

SQUARE stretch

This square position opens your lower spine and releases your hip joints and legs where they connect to your pelvis. This in turn creates space for movement.

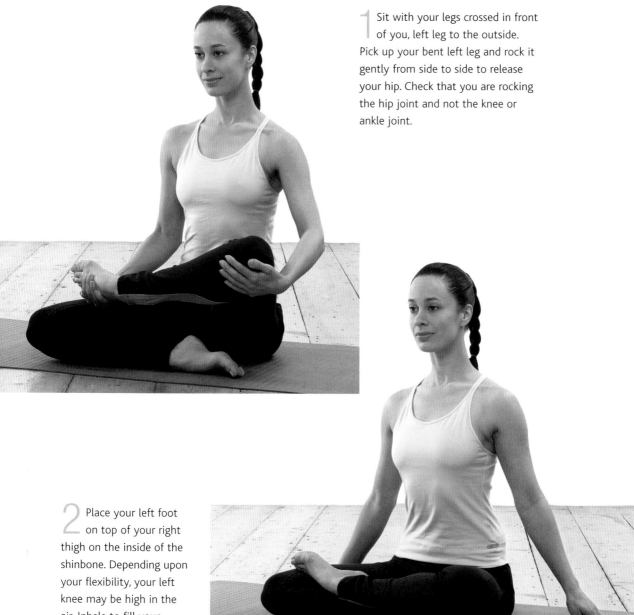

1 Sit with your legs crossed in front of you, left leg to the outside. Pick up your bent left leg and rock it gently from side to side to release your hip. Check that you are rocking the hip joint and not the knee or ankle joint.

2 Place your left foot on top of your right thigh on the inside of the shinbone. Depending upon your flexibility, your left knee may be high in the air. Inhale to fill your ribcage and as you exhale, lengthen upwards through your spine.

3 Inhale and, as you exhale, extend your arms in front of you and allow your trunk to bend forwards over your legs. **Hold for 1–3 minutes,** then repeat on the other side.

stretch

SPINE stimulation

This stretch stimulates all the muscles along your spinal column and helps to increase movement in your hips and legs. It also stimulates blood circulation to the organs found in the abdominal area such as the stomach, liver and kidneys. As you do this exercise keep your neck long to maximize the benefit.

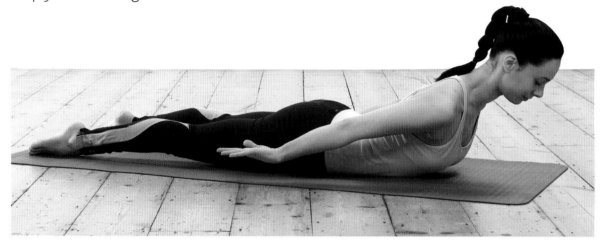

1 Lie on your stomach with your arms at your sides. Inhale and raise your head, chest and arms up as high as is comfortable. Exhale and draw your abdomen in towards your spine to protect your back muscles.

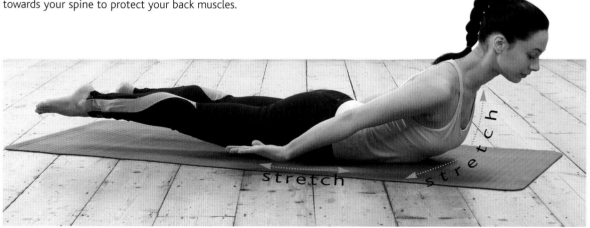

2 Inhale to fill your ribcage and, as you exhale, gently raise your legs a short distance off the floor. Keep your lower back soft and your chest open. Allow your body to decide how high you can lift. **Hold for 5 breath cycles,** then exhale as you lower your legs and chest.

SPINE arch

This posture works to re-establish the natural lumbar curve of the spine that is lost through sitting for hours. This is a strong, effective stretch that helps to open the area of the spine that is tight in most people. If you have a back problem that prevents you flattening your back, then this exercise is not suitable for you.

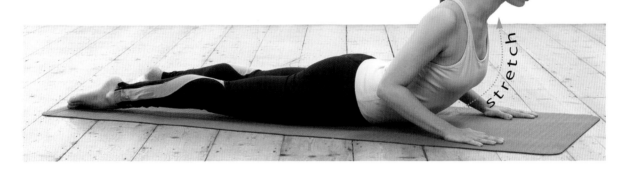

1 Lie on your stomach with your hands on the floor level with your shoulders. Turn your hands slightly so your fingers are pointing out a little. Relax your pelvic floor. Inhale and lift your ribcage up, keeping your elbows soft, so your stomach and pelvis are suspended above the floor.

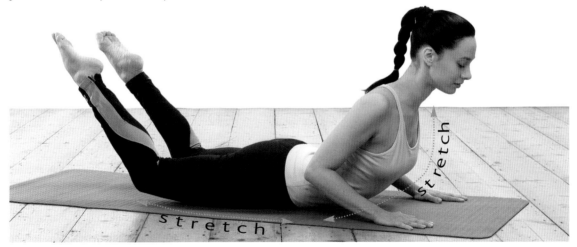

2 Exhale and relax into the stretch. Inhale to fill your ribcage and, as you exhale, lengthen your abdomen and lift your feet off the floor towards the ceiling. **Hold for 10–15 breath cycles.**

EASY back STRETCH

Also known as the Child's pose, this stretch gently relaxes your spine, especially after doing back bends. It also inclines your head so your heart can rest instead of trying to force blood up to your brain.

1 Start on your hands and knees with your hands under your shoulders and your knees under your hips.

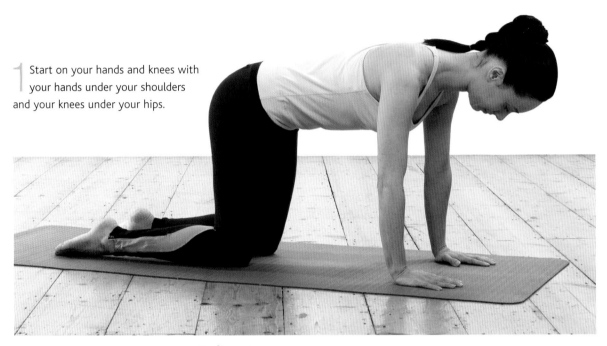

stretch

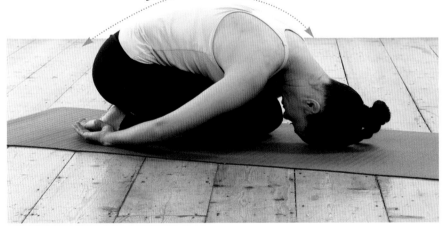

2 Inhale into your ribcage and, as you exhale, sit back on your heels. Place your head on the floor and your arms, one by one, to your sides. Invite relaxation into the whole of your body. Close your eyes and empty your mind. **Hold for 1–2 minutes.**

SPINE twist

A great stretch that releases any tension from your tailbone (sacrum) area, opens your hips and frees your pelvis. If you manage to do this stretch every day, you will really feel the benefit in your back.

1 Lie on your back with your legs extended and your arms by your sides. Inhale and draw your left knee in towards your left shoulder. Exhale and draw your abdomen in towards your spine.

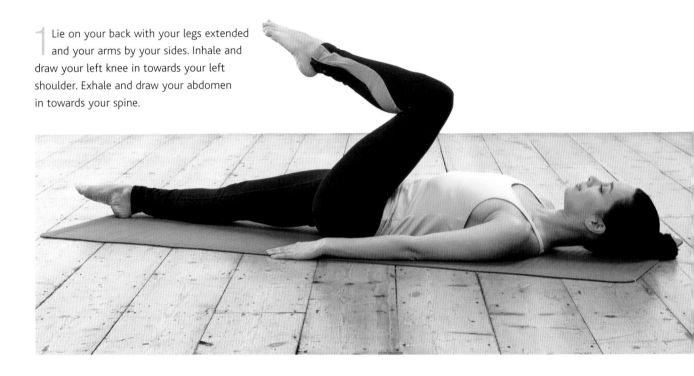

2 Place your right hand on the outside of your left knee and place your left arm on the floor in line with your right shoulder. Inhale and, as you exhale, draw your left knee over to the right. Keep your shoulders on the floor. **Hold for 10 breath cycles,** then repeat on the other side.

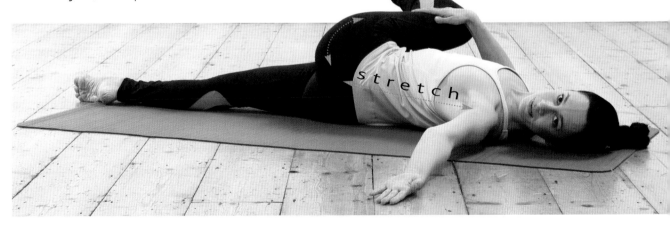

stretch

CROSS-LEG forward BEND

Another effective stretch that releases your spine and knees and can be done every day. This technique releases tensions from the outer hip sockets and softens any tension in the spine.

1 Sit with your legs crossed, with your left leg on the inside and your right leg on the outside. Lift up through your spine and lengthen your abdomen.

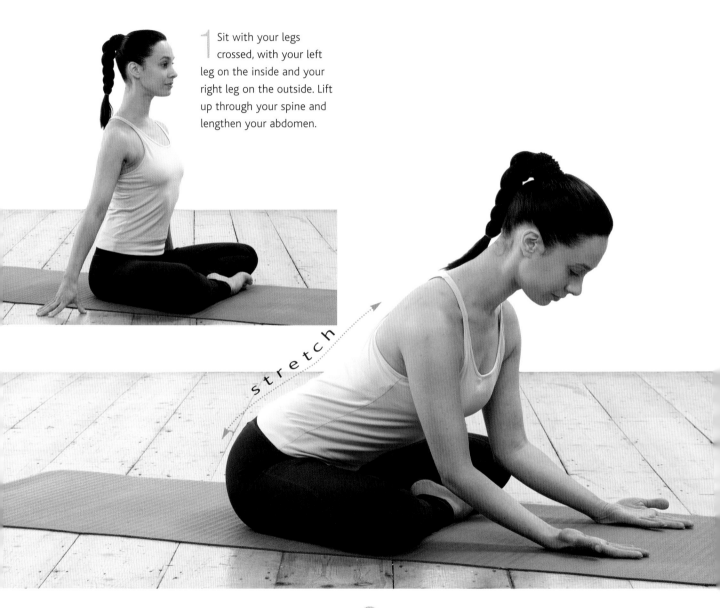

stretch

2 Inhale to fill your ribcage and, as you exhale, move your arms in front of you and allow your chest to extend over your legs, releasing the spine. Try not to drop your chest and aim to maintain space in your lungs and ribcage. **Hold for 1–5 minutes.** Cross your legs the other way and repeat.

SUPINE leg STRETCH

There are three stages to this stretch, so work to your own level. The stretches are designed to target your hamstring muscles, spine and legs; breathe deeply throughout to release tension from these areas.

TIP

When stretching, aim to keep your spine in a 'neutral' position, which means that it does not move, arch or curve as you move. This helps to protect and strengthen your back and abdominal muscles.

1 Lie on your back with both knees bent. Inhale and draw your right leg upwards and towards your chest. Exhale and hold your calf or the back of your thigh. Inhale and, as you exhale, lengthen your left foot away from you while maintaining a neutral spine.

stretch

stretch

2 Inhale to fill your ribcage and, as you exhale, reach up with your trunk and hold your big toe with your first two fingers. Relax your trunk back towards the floor. With your spine now long on the floor, draw your right thigh muscle onto your right thighbone and draw your leg towards your chest again. **Hold for 10–15 breath cycles.**

VARIATION

Aim to extend your extended leg out to your side and flat along the floor as your flexibility develops.

stretch

SUPINE thigh STRETCH

This version of the lying stretch helps to relax your outer thighs and opens your hip joints. This helps to release your lumbar spine.

1 Lie on your back with both knees bent. Inhale and exhale to draw your right leg towards your chest. Inhale to fill your ribcage and, as you exhale, lengthen the left foot away from you while maintaining a neutral spine.

2 Inhale and reach up to hold your big toe with the first two fingers of your left hand. Exhale and release your right arm along the floor keeping your arm in line with your shoulder.

3 Inhale to fill your ribcage and, as you exhale, draw your right leg across your body without tilting your pelvis. Keep your shoulders on the floor. **Hold for 15 breath cycles.** Repeat on the other side.

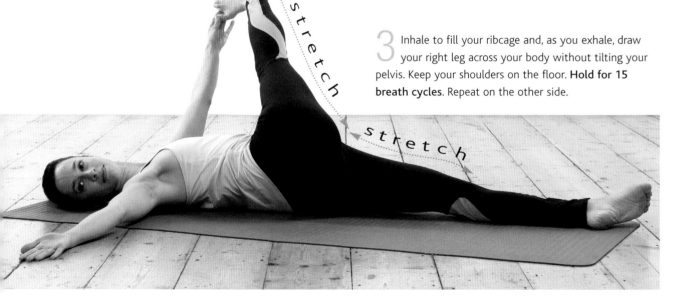

SUPINE groin STRETCH

This version of the lying stretch targets your groin area and helps to stretch the deep muscles that originate in your lumbar spine and go into the pelvic floor muscle. This stretch also helps to strengthen your abdominals.

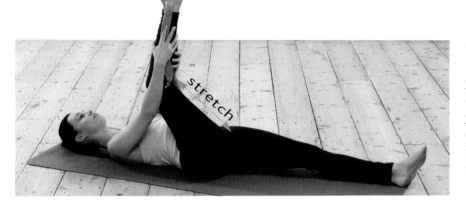

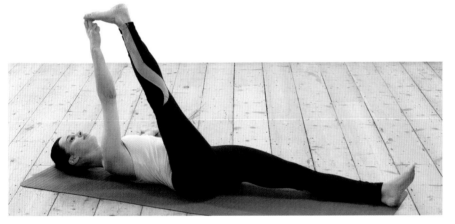

1 Lie on your back. Inhale and exhale to draw your right leg towards your chest. Inhale again to fill your ribcage and, as you exhale, lengthen your left foot away from you while maintaining a neutral spine.

2 Inhale and place your left arm on the floor in line with your left shoulder. Hold the big toe of your right foot with the first two fingers of your right hand.

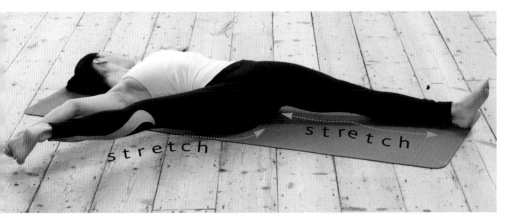

3 Inhale to fill your ribcage and, as you exhale, take your right leg out to the side keeping your left hip on the floor. Draw your abdomen into your spine to stabilize your body. **Hold for 10–15 breath cycles**, then repeat on the other side.

ROCKING stretch

A great massage for the connective tissue that links your lower spine and groin areas. It also encourages circulation, which helps to lubricate tight joints and stiff muscles.

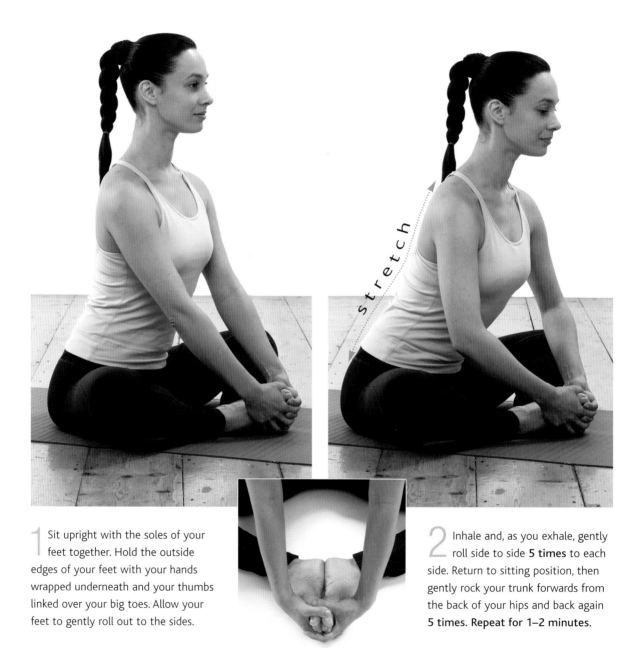

stretch

1 Sit upright with the soles of your feet together. Hold the outside edges of your feet with your hands wrapped underneath and your thumbs linked over your big toes. Allow your feet to gently roll out to the sides.

2 Inhale and, as you exhale, gently roll side to side **5 times** to each side. Return to sitting position, then gently rock your trunk forwards from the back of your hips and back again **5 times. Repeat for 1–2 minutes.**

WIDE plough STRETCH

A great technique for opening your groin area and neck, as well as deeply stretching along the length of your spine.

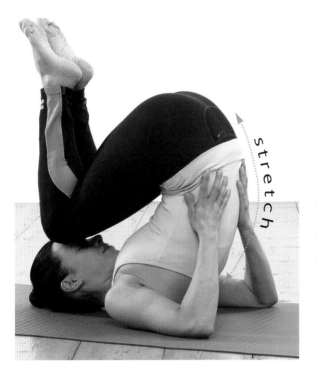

1 Lie on your back with your knees bent towards your chest and your palms resting on your lower back. Inhale and, as you exhale, push your abdomen and hands upwards so your knees rest on your forehead. **Hold for 1–3 breath cycles.**

2 Inhale and, as you exhale, extend your legs over your head to place the balls of your feet firmly on the floor. Open your legs into a wide plough position. Keep your shoulders open and broad. **Hold for 1–4 minutes.**

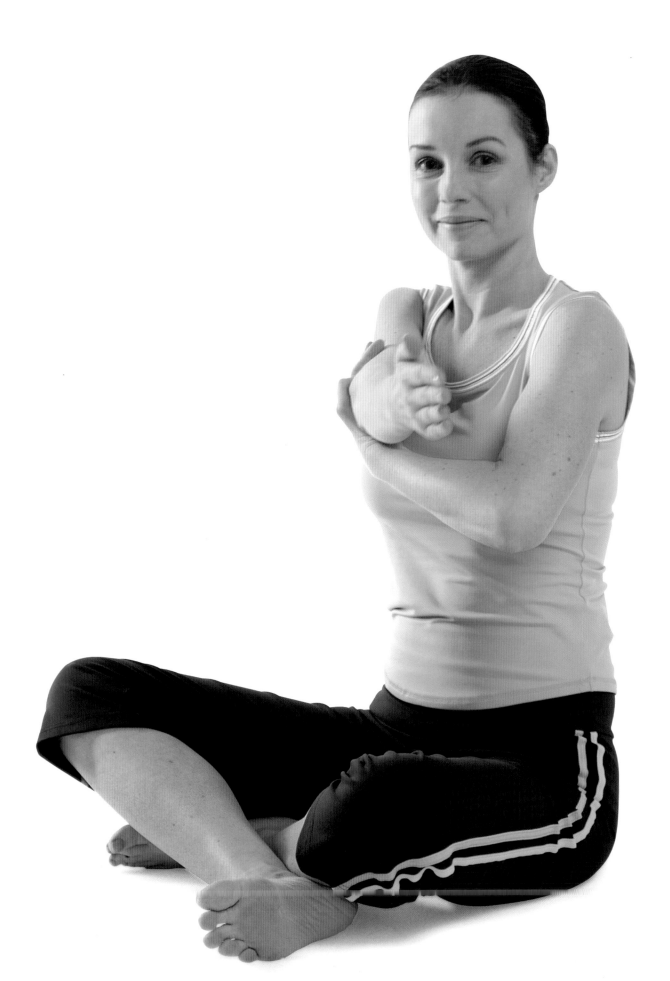

STRETCHING YOUR UPPER BODY

The stretches in this section will help to ease the strains and stresses that collect in the upper body. Most of us are familiar with the tension that can collect around the neck and shoulders due to daily tasks such as typing on a keyboard or carrying children. Discomfort and pain can build in the upper body and manifest itself in headaches or debilitating shoulder and neck pain.

Releasing the tension from your neck, shoulders and upper spine will really improve your wellbeing. These stretches will also create more space between the tiny vertebrae of the spine found towards the neck. This can improve your upper body posture, which is especially important as this is an area of your body people notice most.

Perform the movements slowly and take care in particular when mobilizing your neck; avoid any sudden or jarring movements.

THIS SECTION INCLUDES 10 UPPER BODY SUPER STRETCHES:

SEATED neck SPACER

Moving and stretching your neck is important to maintain length in the sides of your neck. This stretch helps to prevent or alleviate headaches and any stiffness in your shoulders.

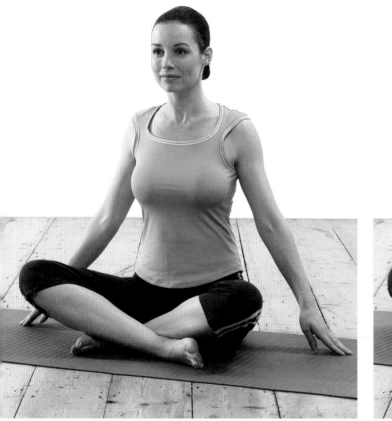

stretch

1 Sit with your legs crossed and your arms resting at your sides. Inhale and lengthen your spine.

2 Rest your left hand on the right-hand side of your head. Exhale and draw your left ear towards your left shoulder, keeping your shoulders level. Slowly return to centre and repeat on the other side. **Repeat 10 times, slowly in time with your breath.** Each time aim to deepen the range of movement.

VARIATION

If you find sitting with your legs crossed uncomfortable, sit in any other comfortable position, for example, on a firm, supportive chair.

CAUTION

When mobilizing your neck, work slowly and with care; do not rush or force the movement.

SEATED neck STRETCH

This stretch focuses on the central neck muscles. If you practise this stretch regularly, it can help to improve your posture and give you more length in your neck.

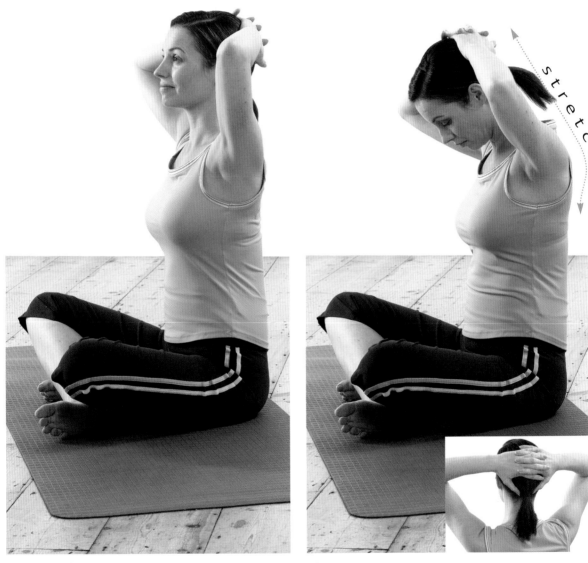

1 Sit with your legs crossed or in any other comfortable position. Inhale and raise your arms to place your palms on the side of your head with your fingers touching at the back. Be careful not to push; the weight of your arms will be enough.

2 Exhale and gently draw your chin down towards your chest. **Hold for 5 breath cycles.** Gently unclasp your hands and allow your arms to come out of position. Curl your head up gently. **Repeat 5 times.**

SHOULDER release

A great way to release tension from around your shoulder joints.
This can help to increase mobility and relieve aches following sport
or working at a desk.

1 Sit with your legs crossed or in any other position that is comfortable for you.

2 Inhale and bring your right arm across your chest towards your left. Exhale and place your left hand on to the outside of your right upper arm, then apply a little pressure to bring the arm across further and to ease open the shoulder joint. **Hold for 5 breath cycles. Repeat on both sides 3 times.**

stretch

UPPER arm STRETCH

This stretches the triceps muscles found in the backs of your arms. It is very useful to relieve arm tiredness after carrying children or weight training, for example.

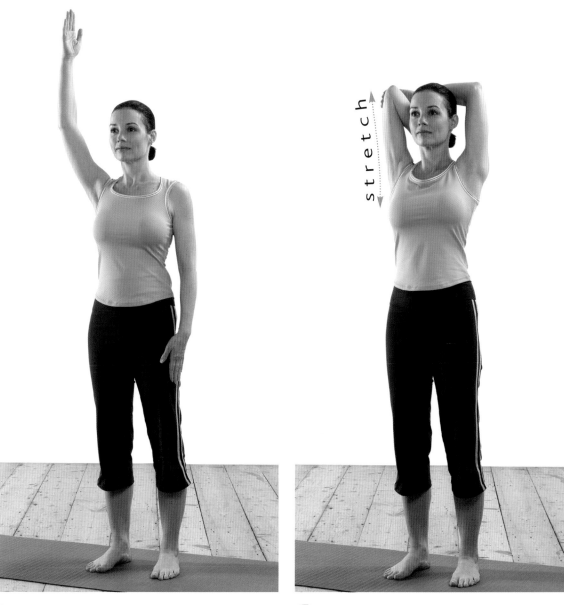

1 Stand with your feet hip-width apart. Inhale to fill your ribcage and extend your right arm into the air in line with your right shoulder.

2 Exhale and drop your right hand down between your shoulder blades. Inhale and take your left hand to your right elbow and exhale, applying a little pressure to lengthen the triceps muscle. **Hold for 5 breath cycles and repeat 3 times on each side.**

SEATED chest STRETCH

A great stretch for releasing your breath, offsetting depression and opening your chest muscles.

1 Sit with your legs crossed, with your spine long and your buttock bones grounded to the floor. Inhale and take your hands behind you as far as is comfortable. Exhale and roll onto the palms of your hands.

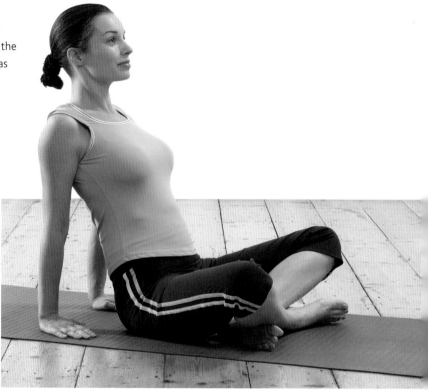

stretch

2 Inhale to fill your ribcage and, as you exhale, lift your sternum and ribcage up and backwards. Lengthen through your ribcage. **Hold for 5 breath cycles, then release. Repeat 5 times,** aiming to deepen the range of movement each time.

WRIST stretch

If you work with your hands, this is a very good stretch to help offset repetitive strain injury. Try to remember to do this throughout the day, especially after long periods of working with your hands.

1 Sit with your legs stretched out in a straddle position. Inhale and lengthen through your spine keeping your buttock bones on the floor. Exhale, engage your abdomen muscles and draw them in towards your spine.

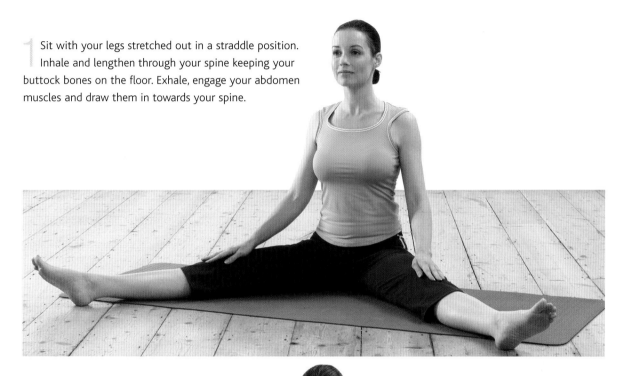

2 Place the backs of your hands on the floor in front of you, shoulder-width apart, with your fingers pointing up towards you. Inhale and, as you exhale, gently press down on your hands feeling the stretch in your wrist. **Hold for 5 breath cycles, then repeat 5 times.**

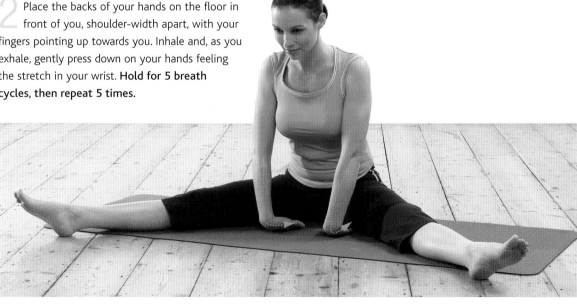

SEATED waist STRETCH

This technique lengthens your spine, hips and waist as well as warming your lungs and the supporting breathing muscles.

1 Sit with your legs crossed and with your spine lengthened. Inhale and raise your right arm upwards.

2 As you exhale, reach your right arm over your head to the left, bending from the waist as you slide your left palm away on the floor. Keep your hand grounded and your elbow soft. **Hold for 5 breath cycles**, then repeat on the other side.

stretch

CHEST release

This stretch helps to release any tension you feel around your chest and shoulders areas. Tightness in the chest area can lead to round shoulders and poor posture, which can feel uncomfortable and restrict breathing.

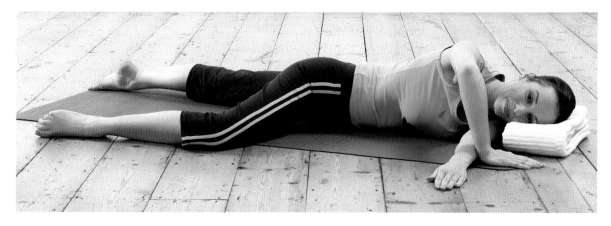

1 Lie on your front with your feet hip-width apart. Place your left arm under your chest and out to your right side in line with your shoulder, with your palm facing down. Place your right hand above your left arm, with your elbow pointing upwards. Bring your right knee up in line with your right hip.

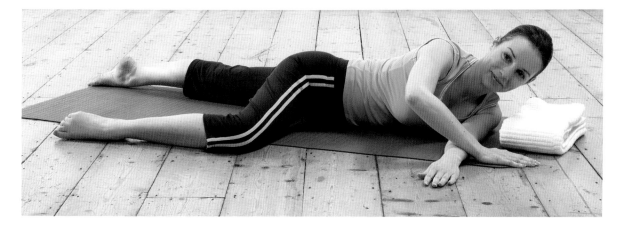

2 Inhale and, as you exhale, gently lift the left side of your upper body away from the floor opening your shoulder joint. Keep your head in line with your spine and be careful not to drop your hip forward. **Hold for 5 breath cycles. Repeat 2 times on each side.**

FORWARD release

A great stretch for opening the front of your shoulders and releasing tension in your neck and spine.

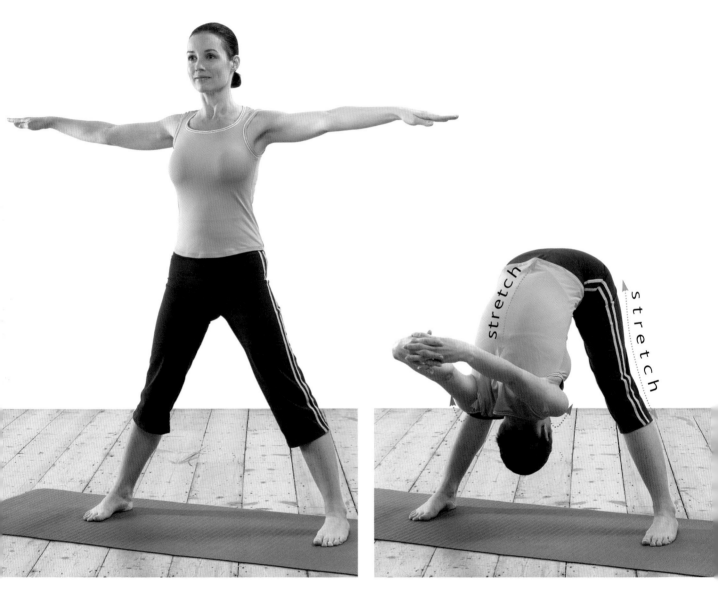

1 Stand with your feet as wide as you can, arms out to your sides. Lift your hip bones and lengthen your tailbone. Inhale to fill your ribcage. At the same time raise your arms out to your sides until they are shoulder height. Exhale and lengthen your abdomen.

2 Inhale, and as you exhale, clasp your hands together behind your back. Inhale and as you exhale, bend your knees slightly and hinge forwards at your hips, allowing your arms to stretch over your head. **Hold for 5 breath cycles.** Inhale and, as you exhale, draw in your abdomen to support you as you stand up slowly.

HEAD roll

A lovely softener to release tension from around your brain and skull. It is a great stretch for offsetting headaches, so aim to repeat it throughout the day, especially if you are working.

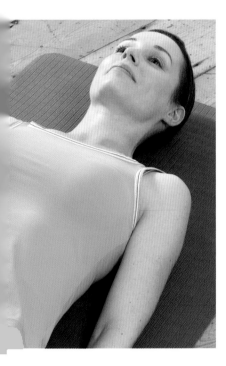 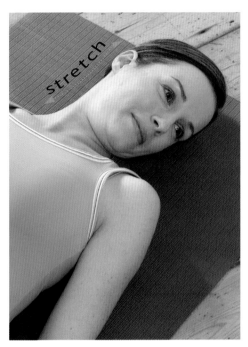 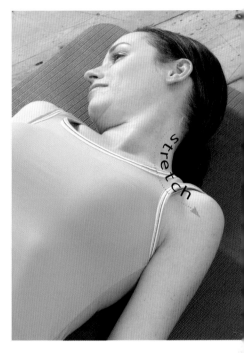

1 Lie on your back with your knees bent and your arms resting by the sides of your body with your palms facing upwards. Check that your spine feels comfortable.

2 Press your chin gently in towards your chest to lengthen the back of your neck. Inhale and, as you exhale, press the back of your head into the floor and turn it about 30 degrees to the left. **Hold for 1 breath cycle.**

3 Inhale and take your head back to the centre. As you exhale, repeat to the right side. **Hold for 1 breath cycle. Repeat each side 5 times** aiming to increase the rotation on each turning of your head.

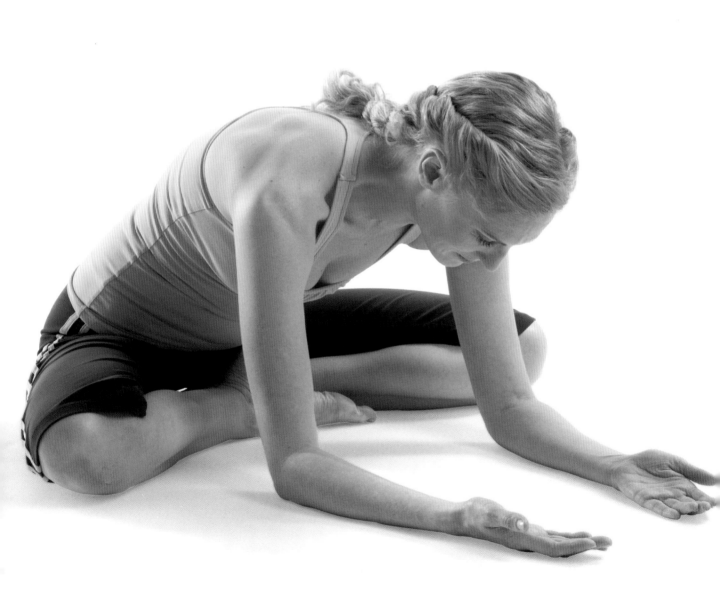

GENTLE THERAPEUTIC STRETCHES

Use this section if you don't have much energy, but want to do a gentle stretch routine that targets the connective tissue that links your muscles to your bones. These stretches can help to alleviate aches and pains and energize you. They also massage and stimulate your vital organs, as well as allowing more space for the organs to function properly. This section does not require much energy but it will be a little uncomfortable as you open your joints softly.

As we age, the tissue that connects our muscles and bones can become dry and brittle, as fluids decrease within our bodies. Stretching and moving your joints helps to increase the flow of cerebral spinal fluid around the body. This fluid carries serotonin and other hormones that can help to lift your mood and make your body feel good.

Stretching your joints is not always a comfortable journey as you may have been collecting tension for many years; it will take a little time for your joints to respond and soften. The stretches in this section will help you to recognize the 'letting go' zone in each stretch – the point at which you relax and let your muscles lengthen.

THIS SECTION INCLUDES 12 GENTLE SUPER STRETCHES:

- Seated straddle (see page 112)
- Trunk over leg (see page 113)
- Child's pose (see page 114)
- Pigeon hip roll (see page 115)
- Splits pelvis roll (see page 116)
- Forward bend (see page 117)
- Seated cross-leg bend (see page 118)
- Extended square stretch (see page 119)
- Shoelace forward bend (see page 120)
- Shoelace circles (see page 121)
- Liver roll (see page 122)
- Figure of 8 roll (see page 123)

SEATED straddle

This stretch softens the connective tissue surrounding your inner and outer hip sockets. It also massages your liver and kidneys as you move around the stretch.

TIP

Let your body tell you where the tension is and, as long as it is comfortable, focus your movements around this area. As you exhale during the movement, zone in on the spot that gives you the most obvious sensations, whether these are pleasurable or uncomfortable, and relax there.

1 Sit on the floor with your legs stretched out in a straddle position, with your spine long. Inhale and, as you exhale, allow your trunk to hinge forwards at your hips until you feel a light stretch up the backs of your legs, hips and back.

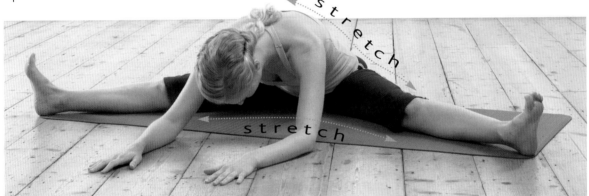

2 Inhale to fill your ribcage and, as you exhale, allow your body to gently move around the straddle position to your right, walking your hands along the floor. Explore the changing sensations that happen in your body. **Continue for 1–3 minutes,** then repeat in the other direction.

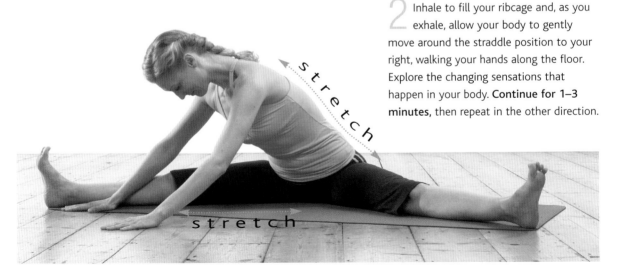

VARIATION

If you need to give your spine a rest before changing to the other side, roll down slowly onto your back and bring your knees in towards your chest. This releases your back.

TRUNK over LEG

This technique is a variation on the previous stretch but it targets the sides of your waist. It also massages the intestines, kidneys and liver organs and really feels great.

1 Sit on the floor with your legs stretched in a straddle position and your sitting bones grounded fully to the floor. Inhale and lengthen through your spine. Rest your left hand on your left thigh and stretch your right arm along the inside of your right leg. Exhale.

s t r e t c h

2 Inhale and lift your left arm upwards over your head to deepen the stretch in the side of your trunk and spine. Exhale and relax. **Hold for 1–3 minutes, keeping your breath natural.** Repeat on the other side.

s t r e t c h

s t r e t c h

CHILD'S pose

This technique gently massages your liver and softens the connective tissue around your hip sockets. It also helps to create space between the discs in your spine.

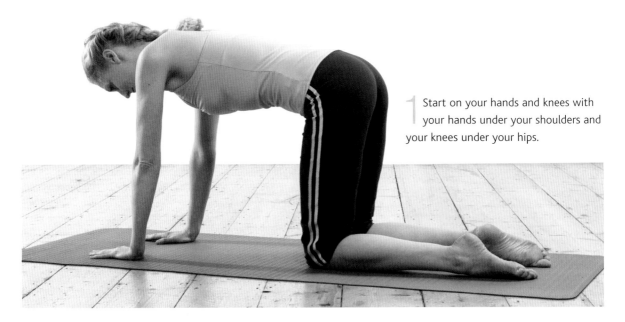

1 Start on your hands and knees with your hands under your shoulders and your knees under your hips.

2 Inhale into your ribcage and, as you exhale, sit back onto your heels. Rest your forehead on the floor. Focus on letting go of any tension in your pelvis and spine. Inhale and, as you exhale, begin to shift your pelvis from side to side, gently moving around the central axis of the stretch. **Do this slowly for 2–3 minutes.**

s t r e t c h

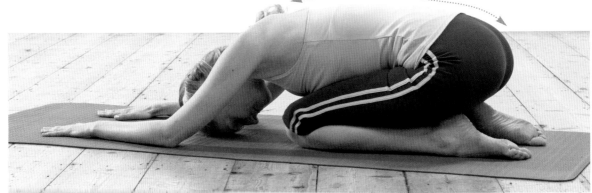

PIGEON hip ROLL

This stretch works to increase essential fluids to your hip area, helping to soften problem areas around the hips and pelvis.

TIP

Focus your movements around any area of tension. As you exhale, zone in on the spot that gives you the most obvious sensations, whether these are pleasurable or uncomfortable.

1 Start on your hands and knees in the box position. Place your left knee between your hands and extend your right leg away behind you. Lift your spine.

2 Inhale and roll onto your left buttock bone. As you exhale, roll onto the outside of your right hip moving your hands to where it is comfortable.

3 Continue to move from side to side, gradually lowering and extending your hands and ribcage forwards until you can rest your forehead on your hands. **Spend 1–2 minutes rolling,** then repeat on the other side.

SPLITS pelvis ROLL

This stretch softens your hip sockets and helps to make the splits position feel lighter and easier; the movement distracts you from any feelings of discomfort you might experience. You need to be sensitive to your body to improve in this stretch.

1 Start by kneeling on the floor. Place your left foot forwards and extend your right leg behind you. Place your hands or fingertips on the floor for support. Inhale and, as you exhale, press your hips forwards into the 'splits' position (see page 80). Extend your spine and move your hands to where it is comfortable.

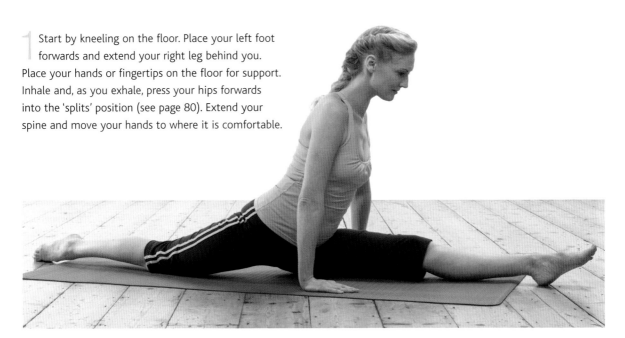

2 Exhale and slowly roll your pelvis side to side as you lower your ribcage towards your thighs, bringing your elbows towards the floor. Pause if the sensations become painful. Your breathing will speed up when you touch an area of chronic tension. It's important to breathe and find a comfortable, not painful, place to rest. **Roll for 1–2 minutes.** Come out of the position gently and change sides.

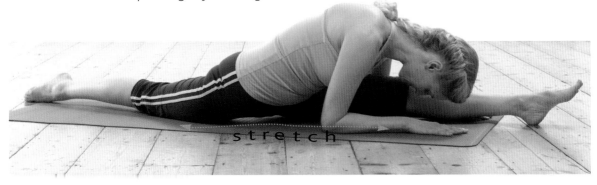

stretch

FORWARD bend

This variation of the Seated forward bend (see page 50) introduces a rocking movement that promotes more fluid circulating around your lumbar spine and legs.

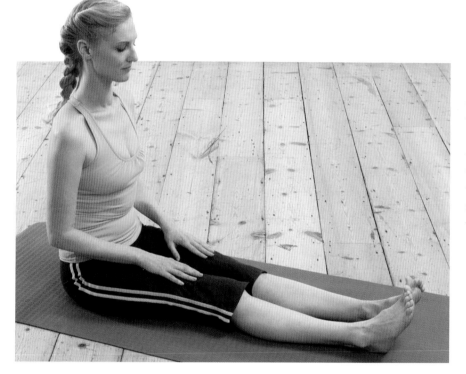

1 Sit upright with your legs stretched in front of you. Press your legs together so your ankles, inner calves and thighs touch. Roll your shin and thigh bones softly in towards one another to release any locking in your tailbone area (sacrum).

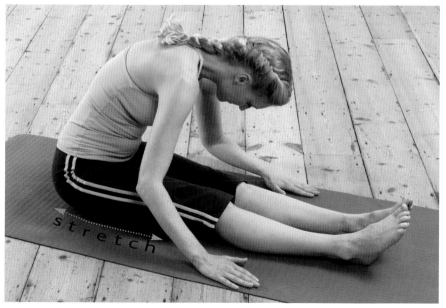

2 Place your hands by the sides of your legs. Inhale and, as you exhale, allow your trunk to move softly from side to side, gently lengthening it forwards towards your thighs. Keep your buttocks on the floor. **Continue rolling for 1–2 minutes,** maintaining an open chest and long spine.

SEATED cross-leg BEND

An easy stretch that helps to soften the connective tissue around your lower spine and pelvis. It also helps to optimize organ function by massaging the kidneys, liver and pancreas, while pacifying the adrenal glands.

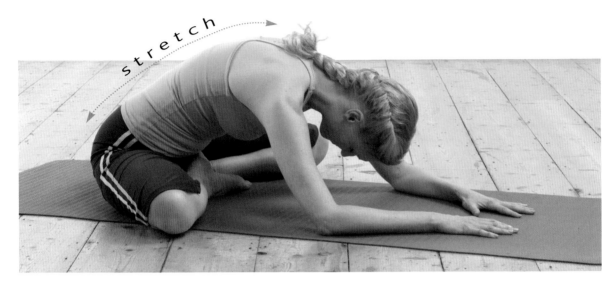

1 Sit with your legs crossed with your left leg on the inside and your right leg on the outside. Inhale and lengthen through your spine. As you exhale, allow your ribcage and arms to extend forwards to lengthen your spine.

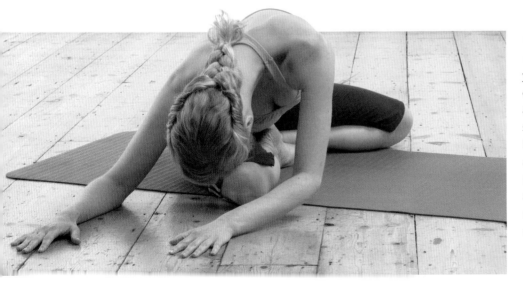

2 Inhale and, as you exhale, begin to move your trunk to the right in a circular movement, being aware of the changing sensations in your hips, back and legs. Find the area where you feel the most obvious sensations and **rest there for 1–2 minutes.** Repeat on the other side.

EXTENDED SQUARE stretch

Once you find the Seated cross-leg bend straightforward, progress to this exercise to feel the stretch on a deeper level. This stretch can help to open the kidneys and pacify the adrenal glands.

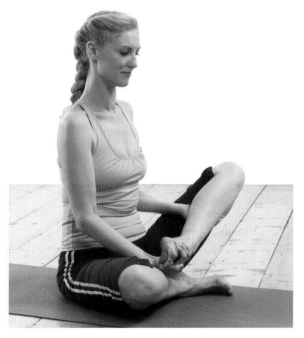

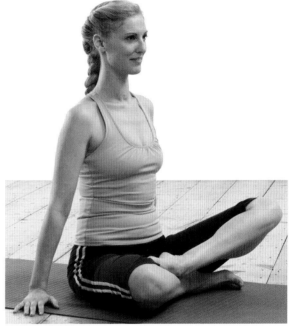

1 Sit with your legs crossed in front of you. Pick up your bent left leg and rock it gently from side to side to release your hip. Check that you are rocking your hip joint and not your knee or ankle joint, and that your right ankle is square to your left knee.

2 Place your left foot on top of your right inner calf. Depending upon your flexibility, your left knee may be high in the air. Inhale to fill your ribcage and as you exhale, lengthen upwards through your spine.

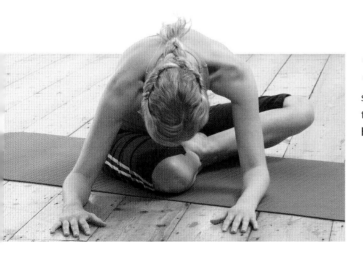

3 Inhale and, as you exhale, move your hips and ribcage around the square position exploring all the changing sensations in your body. Slowly lower your trunk towards the floor. **Find where you feel the stretch the most and hold for 1–3 minutes.** Repeat on the other side.

SHOELACE forward BEND

This stretch helps to soften and open your lower back. It also massages your adrenal glands and is a great softener for the connective tissue that links your legs to your pelvis.

TIP

This can be quite an uncomfortable stretch if your hips are stiff, so work gently and aim to increase the time spent in the position by 30 seconds each time.

1 Start on your hands and knees with your hands under your shoulders and your knees under your hips. Cross your legs over so the left leg is behind the right.

VARIATION
If you can bend towards the floor, curl your hands into fists, and rest your head on your hands for support.

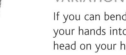
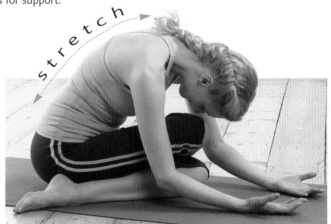
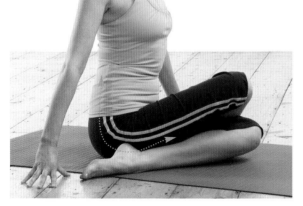

2 Open your feet and sit down in the space between your feet. Ensure both sitting bones are grounded and your spine is long. Place your hands on the floor. Inhale to lengthen through your spine then, as you exhale, lengthen your abdomen. Sit in this position for 1–3 minutes

3 Inhale and, as you exhale, allow your trunk to extend forwards. Inhale and, as you exhale, relax further into a soft forward bend. Hold the stretch at the threshold of feeling uncomfortable. Keep your ribcage open and your abdomen long and empty. Hold for 2–4 minutes.

SHOELACE circles

This technique is a variation on the Shoelace forward bend opposite. It helps to soften the connective tissue around your outer thighs and hip sockets. It also massages the intestines, aiding digestion.

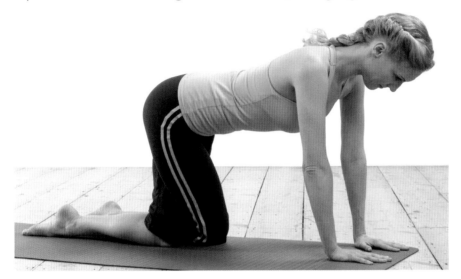

1 Start on your hands and knees with your hands under your shoulders and your knees under your hips. Cross your legs over so the left leg is behind the right.

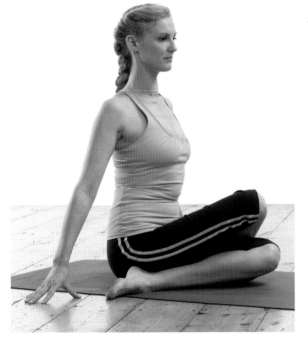

2 Open your feet and sit down in the space between your feet. Ensure both sitting bones are grounded and your spine is long. Place your hands on the floor.

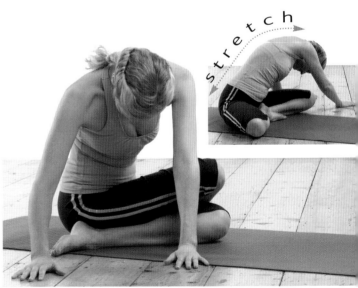

3 Inhale and fill out your ribcage. As you exhale, walk your hands around to the right bringing your trunk into a small twist and opening the left side of your back. **Hold for 1–3 minutes,** then repeat on the other side.

LIVER roll

A great massage for your liver, helping to detoxify your blood supply. It also pacifies the pancreas that is responsible for controlling your blood sugar and hormone levels. The deep breathing releases the toxins out of your body.

TIP

Aim to make your circles bigger and heavier with each breath cycle. This will increase the range of movement throughout your body.

1 Lie on your back with your feet flat on the floor. Bring your knees into your chest and wrap your hands around them. Inhale and, as you exhale, roll your knees in a clockwise direction to massage the lumbar spine. **Repeat 5 times,** then repeat in the other direction.

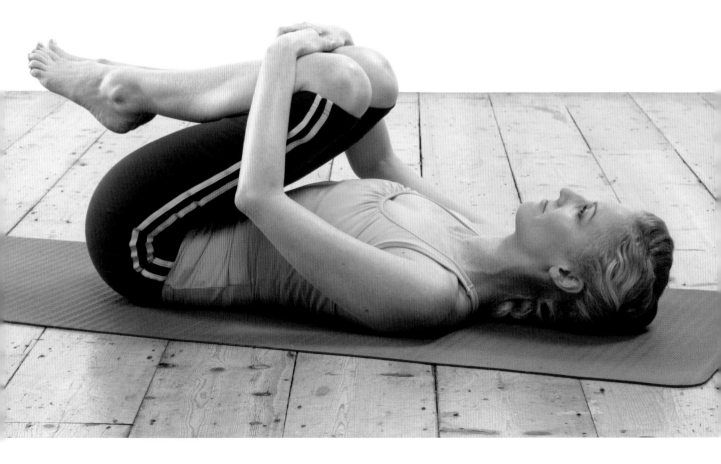

FIGURE of 8 roll

A variation on the Liver roll, this stretch encourages a real 'feel-good' massage around your spine and hips. It works through the full range of hip movement, so enjoy it and work slowly.

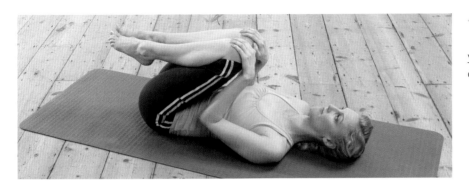

1 Lie on your back with your knees bent and your hands resting gently on your knees.

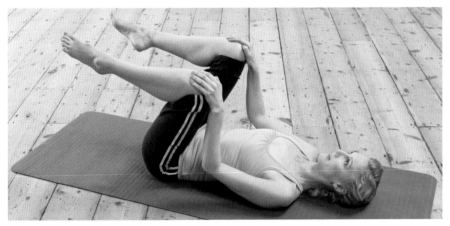

2 Inhale and, as you exhale, raise your right knee gently, keeping both hands on your knees for support. Inhale and, as you exhale, circle your right leg in a clockwise direction, rolling slightly to your right onto the rear part of your pelvis. This is a circular motion for both your hips and legs.

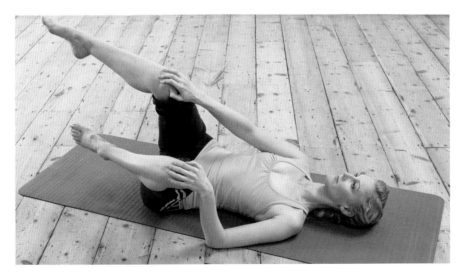

3 Inhale and, as you exhale, circle your leg to the left side of your pelvis, drawing a 'figure of 8' with your knees. **Repeat slowly 15 times,** then repeat with the other leg.

CAUTION

If you feel any clunking or grinding in your hips move very slowly to help ease stiffness. If you experience any pain, stop immediately and see a physiotherapist for advice.

INDEX

ACKNOWLEDGEMENTS

The author

Jax Lysycia is a half-share Director of Dynamic Yoga Teacher Training UK, training Yoga Teachers with Godfrey Devereux. She has also pioneered the highly successful FormenteraYoga.com specializing in the coolest Balearic Yoga retreats. Jax has studied Dance and Movement for over 13 years and she still teaches teachers and clients every week in her studio in Essex in the UK. Jax is considered to be one the best yoga/stretch teachers in the world, as voted by *Yoga Magazine* November 2005.

Publisher's acknowledgements

The publisher would like to thank USA Pro for supplying a selection of clothing to use at the photo shoot.

Executive Editor Jane McIntosh
Editor Camilla Davis
Executive Art Director Darren Southern
Designer Janis Utton
Photographer Mike Prior
Artwork Illustrator Sudden Impact Media
Production Manager Nigel Reed

Special photography: Octopus Publishing Group Ltd/Mike Prior